DRUG TRANSIT AND DISTRIBUTION, INTERCEPTION AND CONTROL

FDA's Expedited Drug Programs

Analysis, Postmarket Monitoring and Industry Guidance

DRUG TRANSIT AND DISTRIBUTION, INTERCEPTION AND CONTROL

Additional books in this series can be found on Nova's website under the Series tab.

Additional e-books in this series can be found on Nova's website under the eBooks tab.

DRUG TRANSIT AND DISTRIBUTION, INTERCEPTION AND CONTROL

FDA'S EXPEDITED DRUG PROGRAMS

ANALYSIS, POSTMARKET MONITORING AND INDUSTRY GUIDANCE

GARY LAWRENCE
EDITOR

Novinka
New York

NOTICE TO THE READER

Library of Congress Cataloging-in-Publication Data

ISBN: 978-1-63485-772-7

Published by Nova Science Publishers, Inc. † New York

CONTENTS

PREFACE

The Food and Drug Administration (FDA) oversees the safety and effectiveness of drugs sold on the U.S. market. When there is an unmet need for the treatment of a serious condition, FDA may use one or more of its expedited programs, such as fast track and breakthrough therapy designation, which are intended to bring drugs to market more quickly. FDA is also responsible for monitoring the safety of drugs and reporting on those efforts. This book examines the number and types of requests for fast track or breakthrough therapy designation; the number and types of FDA-approved drug applications that used an expedited program; and the extent to which FDA's data on tracked safety issues and postmarket studies allowed the agency to meet its reporting and oversight responsibilities.

In: FDA's Expedited Drug Programs
Editor: Gary Lawrence
ISBN: 978-1-63485-772-7

Chapter 1

DRUG SAFETY: FDA EXPEDITES MANY APPLICATIONS, BUT DATA FOR POSTAPPROVAL OVERSIGHT NEED IMPROVEMENT*

United States Government Accountability Office

ABBREVIATIONS

BLA	biologic license application
CDER	Center for Drug Evaluation and Research
DARRTS	Document Archiving, Reporting, and Regulatory Tracking System
FDA	Food and Drug Administration
FDAAA	Food and Drug Administration Amendments Act of 2007
HHS	Department of Health and Human Services
NDA	new drug application
NME	new molecular entity

* This is an edited, reformatted and augmented version of The United States Government Accountability Office publication, GAO-16-192, dated December 2015.

WHY GAO DID THIS STUDY

FDA oversees the safety and effectiveness of drugs sold on the U.S. market. When there is an unmet need for the treatment of a serious condition, FDA may use one or more of its expedited programs, such as fast track and breakthrough therapy designation, which are intended to bring drugs to market more quickly. FDA is also responsible for monitoring the safety of drugs and reporting on those efforts.

GAO was asked to provide information about FDA's expedited programs and its postmarket monitoring of expedited and nonexpedited drugs. This report examines (1) the number and types of requests for fast track or breakthrough therapy designation, (2) the number and types of FDA-approved drug applications that used an expedited program, and (3) the extent to which FDA's data on tracked safety issues and postmarket studies allowed the agency to meet its reporting and oversight responsibilities. GAO analyzed FDA data on requests for fast track or breakthrough therapy designation and approved drug applications that used an expedited program from October 1, 2006, to December 31, 2014 (the most recent available). GAO reviewed FDA information on tracked safety issues and postmarket studies, including FDA internal evaluations and guidance, and interviewed FDA officials.

WHAT GAO RECOMMENDS

FDA should develop plans to correct problems with its postmarket safety data and ensure that these data can be easily used for oversight. HHS agreed with GAO's recommendations and provided additional information on FDA's postmarket safety efforts.

WHAT GAO FOUND

From October 1, 2006, to December 31, 2014, the Food and Drug Administration's (FDA) Center for Drug Evaluation and Research (CDER) received about 1,000 requests for fast track designation and breakthrough therapy designation—two of the agency's four expedited programs to facilitate and expedite the development and review of new drugs. Drug sponsors are required to submit formal requests to use these two programs; for the other two expedited programs (accelerated approval and priority review) sponsors are not required to submit formal requests. Regardless of whether sponsors submit a request for an expedited program, they are required to submit a marketing application prior to offering a drug for sale in the United States; using an expedited program does not ensure FDA approval of the marketing application. Sponsors submitted more than 770 requests for fast track designation since fiscal year 2007, and FDA granted about two-thirds of these requests. Sponsors submitted more than 220 requests for breakthrough therapy designation since it was established in July 2012, and the agency denied more than half of these requests.

About a quarter of the drug applications CDER approved for the U.S. market from October 1, 2006, to December 31, 2014, used at least one expedited program, according to FDA data. Included among these applications were new drug applications, biologic license applications, and efficacy supplements, which allow for revisions to the original application, such as changes in the drug's indicated use. Although most of these applications used one program, some applications used two or more, including two oncology drug applications that used all four expedited programs (accelerated approval, breakthrough therapy designation, fast track designation, and priority review). The most common product area among these applications was oncology (19 percent).

FDA lacks reliable, readily accessible data on tracked safety issues and postmarket studies needed to meet certain postmarket safety reporting responsibilities and to conduct systematic oversight. Tracked safety issues are potential safety issues that FDA determines are significant and that it tracks using an internal database. Internal control standards for federal agencies specify that information should be recorded in a form and within a time frame that enables staff to carry out their responsibilities and that relevant, reliable, and timely information should be available for external reporting purposes. However, evaluations conducted by CDER of data in its database revealed problems with the completeness, timeliness, and accuracy of the data. These problems, as well as problems with the way data are recorded that impair their accessibility, have prevented FDA from publishing statutorily required reports on certain potential safety issues and postmarket studies in a timely manner, and have restricted the agency's ability to perform systematic oversight of postmarket drug safety. Although FDA has taken some steps to address the problems with its data, the agency lacks plans that comprehensively outline its efforts and establish related goals and time frames. Additionally, FDA does not have plans to use these data to inform its oversight of its expedited programs, such as determining if drugs that used an expedited program were subsequently associated with tracked safety issues at rates or of types that differed from drugs that used FDA's standard process.

* * *

December 15, 2015

The Honorable Rosa L. DeLauro
Ranking Member
Subcommittee on Labor, Health and Human Services,
Education, and Related Agencies
Committee on Appropriations
House of Representatives

Dear Ms. DeLauro:

The Food and Drug Administration (FDA)—an agency within the Department of Health and Human Services (HHS)—is responsible for overseeing the safety and effectiveness of drugs sold in the United States.[1] Before a drug can be marketed, it must be approved by FDA, which evaluates a drug application to determine whether the new drug is safe and effective for its intended use. While FDA reviews most drug applications using its standard review process, the agency may also utilize one or more of its expedited programs—programs to facilitate and expedite the development and review of new drugs—for drugs that have the potential to address an unmet medical need for the treatment of serious conditions. Although they do not guarantee approval of a marketing application, FDA's expedited programs—accelerated approval, breakthrough therapy designation, fast track designation, and priority review—are intended to reduce the development or review time needed to bring a drug to market. For example, expedited programs may allow for the approval of drugs based on fewer, smaller, or shorter clinical trials. FDA has expressed support for proposals to further streamline the review of certain kinds of drugs, such as antibiotics.[2] However, some patient advocates and researchers have raised questions about whether such efforts could expose patients to drugs that have not been adequately tested and increase the potential for previously unrecognized safety issues to appear once those drugs are more widely used.[3]

Once FDA approves a drug for marketing, whether using an expedited program or not, the agency continues to monitor the drug's safety and is required by law to publicly report on certain aspects of the agency's postmarket safety efforts.[4] For example, FDA identifies and evaluates potential safety issues with marketed drugs, and those that are considered significant are formally tracked in FDA's internal database and referred to as tracked safety issues. FDA also monitors drug sponsors' progress in completing postmarket studies—studies that are conducted after the drug is approved that provide information about a drug's safety, efficacy, or optimal use—that FDA has required or the sponsor has agreed to conduct.[5] However, we and others have found weaknesses in FDA's oversight of postmarket safety for drugs in the past,[6] such as the agency's lack of reliable information to determine the progress of postmarket studies. FDA's use of certain expedited programs to reduce the development time before a drug is approved further increases the importance of the agency's postmarket safety oversight, including the extent to which it is monitoring for unforeseen problems once a drug is on the market.[7]

You asked us to provide information about FDA's use of expedited programs and how FDA monitors the safety of expedited and non-expedited drugs following approval for the U.S. market.[8] This report examines

1. the number and types of requests for fast track or breakthrough therapy designation,
2. the number and types of drug applications that FDA approved for marketing that used one or more expedited programs, and
3. the extent to which FDA's data on tracked safety issues and postmarket studies allowed the agency to meet its reporting and oversight responsibilities.

To examine the number and types of requests for fast track or breakthrough therapy designation, we requested and analyzed data from FDA for these two expedited programs. We focused on the fast track and breakthrough therapy designation programs because drug sponsors are required to submit formal requests to use these two programs; for the other two expedited programs (accelerated approval and priority review) sponsors are not required to submit formal requests.[9] Specifically, we reviewed FDA data on requests for fast track designation and breakthrough therapy designation, and the number of these requests that FDA granted or denied or that were withdrawn by the sponsor. The requests we analyzed were for fast track designation that were received and reviewed by FDA's Center for Drug Evaluation and Research (CDER) from fiscal year 2007 through the first quarter of fiscal year 2015 (the most recent quarter for which data were available at the time of our review), and for breakthrough therapy designation from July 9, 2012, (the date this program was established) through December 31, 2014.[10] The status of the request for fast track or breakthrough therapy designation— such as whether FDA granted or denied the request or if the request was withdrawn by the sponsor—is as of the date that FDA extracted the data we requested.[11] We report data on sponsors' requests for and FDA's decisions about fast track and breakthrough therapy designation by the fiscal year in which the request was made, even if FDA's decision to grant or deny the designation occurred in a subsequent fiscal year. In addition to analyzing the number of requests and the status of FDA's decisions on those requests, we also examined the extent to which requests were granted by FDA product category, which generally corresponds to the FDA review division (e.g., oncology or psychiatry drugs). Requests for fast track and breakthrough therapy designations are generally made before sponsors submit their applications for approval to market a drug, and FDA's decision to grant such a designation does not guarantee that FDA will subsequently approve the application for marketing.

To examine the number and type of drug applications that FDA approved for marketing that used one or more expedited programs, we requested and analyzed data from FDA on all new drug applications (NDA), biologic license applications (BLA), and NDA- and BLA-related efficacy supplements that FDA approved from fiscal year 2007 through the first quarter of fiscal year 2015.[12] We determined the number of applications approved that used FDA's standard process and the number approved that used one or more of FDA's four expedited programs.[13] We also analyzed these data to determine the type of drugs FDA approved, such as the product category.

To examine the extent to which FDA's data on tracked safety issues and postmarket studies allowed the agency to meet its reporting and oversight responsibilities, we requested data from FDA on tracked safety issues and postmarket studies and then interviewed FDA officials tasked with compiling those data.[14] We also reviewed the results of internal evaluations conducted by CDER regarding the quality of the data on tracked safety issues and postmarket studies in the agency's internal database.[15] In addition, we interviewed FDA officials concerning these internal evaluations and their use of data on tracked safety issues and postmarket studies. We assessed FDA's performance against federal internal control standards.[16]

For all three objectives, we reviewed relevant laws and regulations and FDA policy and guidance documents. For our first two objectives, we assessed the reliability of the FDA data by, for example, conducting internal data checks and comparing data FDA provided to us with the agency's publicly available data on drugs approved in a calendar year. We determined that these data were sufficiently reliable for the purposes of this report.

We conducted this performance audit from February 2015 to December 2015 in accordance with generally accepted government auditing standards. Those standards require that we plan and perform the audit to obtain sufficient, appropriate evidence to provide a reasonable basis for our findings and conclusions based on our audit objectives. We believe that the evidence obtained provides a reasonable basis for our findings and conclusions based on our audit objectives.

BACKGROUND

FDA's four expedited programs—accelerated approval, breakthrough therapy designation, fast track designation, and priority review—are intended to facilitate and expedite development and review of new drugs to address unmet medical needs in the treatment of a serious condition.[17]

According to FDA, these programs are intended to help ensure that drugs for serious conditions are approved and available to patients as soon as it can be concluded that the benefits of the drugs justify their risks. Depending on the specific expedited program, sponsors of new drugs may receive a variety of benefits, such as additional opportunities to meet with and obtain advice from FDA officials during drug development; a rolling review—that is, when FDA reviews portions of the application as they come in instead of waiting for the complete application; the ability to use certain surrogate endpoints or an intermediate clinical endpoint that is reasonably likely to predict clinical benefit; or a shorter goal for review time for the drug application.[18] According to FDA, its expedited programs have the potential to shorten the amount of time necessary for a drug to get to market and to reduce development costs for drug sponsors.[19]

There are two different ways that drug applications are selected for review using an expedited program. For breakthrough therapy designation and fast track designation, the sponsor requests and then FDA determines whether to grant or to deny the request, generally during the drug development process before the sponsor submits the application for approval to market the drug.[20] For accelerated approval and priority review, sponsors do not submit formal requests. Instead, discussions between drug sponsors and FDA of the appropriateness of accelerated approval generally begin during the drug development process. For priority review designation, FDA assesses each new drug application when it is submitted to determine if it should undergo priority review. Additionally, drug applications can use multiple expedited programs. For example, in December 2014, FDA granted accelerated approval for Lynparza, a drug to treat advanced ovarian cancer—and this drug application also received priority review. See table 1 for a summary of FDA's expedited programs.

Table 1. Summary of the Food and Drug Administration's (FDA) Expedited Programs for Drugs

Expedited program	Qualifying criteria	Description
Accelerated approval	·Treats a serious condition and drug sponsor demonstrates that a drug generally provides a meaningful advantage over available therapies, and ·Demonstrates an effect on a surrogate endpoint or an intermediate clinical endpoint that is reasonably likely to predict a drug's clinical benefit.[a]	·Determined as part of the review of the marketing application; sponsors do not submit formal requests for review using this expedited program, but FDA encourages sponsors to communicate regarding a drug's potential for accelerated approval early in drug development. ·Requires postmarket confirmatory studies to verify and describeanticipated effect on irreversible morbidity or mortality or other clinical benefit. ·FDA may withdraw approval of the drug or indication approved under accelerated program if the confirmatory studies fail to verify the clinical benefit or do not demonstrate sufficient clinicalbenefit to justify the risks associated with the drug.
Breakthrough therapy designation	·Intended to treat a serious condition,and drug sponsor demonstrates that a drug may provide substantial improvement compared with other available treatments	·Requested by the sponsor, generally during the drug's development and testing before the sponsor submits an application for approval for marketing. ·Features intensive guidance from FDA on efficient drug development, involvement of senior FDA officials, and a rolling review of application materials. ·FDA can rescind breakthrough therapy

Expedited program	Qualifying criteria	Description
	based on preliminary clinical evidence.	designation if drug no longer meets the qualifying criteria.
Fast track designation	·Intended to treat a serious condition, and drug sponsor provides clinical or nonclinical data that demonstrates a drug's potential to address unmet need, or ·Drug designated as a qualified infectious disease product.[b]	·Requested by the sponsor, generally during the drug's development and testing before the sponsor submits an application for approval for marketing. ·Features increased communication with and guidance from FDA officials and may include a rolling review of application materials. ·FDA can rescind fast track designation if drug no longer meets the qualifying criteria.
Priority review	•Drug treats a serious condition, and, if approved, would provide a significant improvement in safety or effectiveness;cor •Supplemental application for a drug proposes a labeling change based on certain pediatric studies; or •Drug designated as a qualified infectious disease product; or •Drug application submitted with a priority review voucher.	•Determined by FDA when the sponsor submits its drug application for approval for marketing; that is, FDA considers allapplications for priority review and it does not require the sponsor to request it. •Reduces goal for taking action on a drug application from 10 months to 6 months.

Source: GAO summary of FDA information. | GAO-16-192.

[a] For accelerated approval, a surrogate endpoint is a laboratory measure or physical sign that is reasonably likely to predict clinical benefit, but is not itself a measure of clinical benefit. For example, tumor shrinkage in certain cancer types has been considered reasonably likely to predict an improvement in overall survival. Similarly, for this expedited program, an intermediate clinical endpoint is a measurement of a therapeutic effect that can be measured earlier than an effect on

irreversible morbidity or mortality and is considered reasonably likely to predict the drug's effect on irreversible morbidity or mortality or other clinical benefit. A clinical endpoint is a direct measure of how a patient feels, functions, or survives.

[b] A drug may be designated as a qualified infectious disease product if it is an antibacterial or antifungal drug intended to treat serious or life-threatening infections.

[c] According to FDA, prior to June 25, 2013, drug applications could qualify for priority review even if the drug product was not intended to treat a serious condition.

FDA has acknowledged that expediting drug application approvals can pose risks for patients. For example, for accelerated approval, FDA guidance states that there is a risk that patients may be exposed to a drug that ultimately will not be shown to provide an actual clinical benefit.[21] FDA's guidance also states that with fewer, smaller, or shorter clinical trials, there may be less information about rare or delayed adverse events. FDA has stated, however, that its expedited programs do not change the standard of evidence required for approval and that some additional risk may be acceptable because patients and physicians are generally willing to accept greater risk when treating life-threatening and severely debilitating diseases.[22]

After FDA approves a drug for marketing, the agency continues to monitor the drug's safety and is required by law to publicly report on certain aspects of its postmarket safety efforts. For example, FDA tracks information about certain potential safety issues, such as serious adverse events and medication errors, in its internal database, the Document Archiving, Reporting, and Regulatory Tracking System (DARRTS).[23] DARRTS is used, among other things, to generate a work plan and assign responsibilities for managing these tracked safety issues, as well as to provide updates on their status. Only those potential safety issues that FDA determines are significant—that is, have the potential to result in FDA taking one or more actions, such as requiring labeling changes—are tracked in DARRTS. FDA is required to publish a quarterly report listing certain potential safety issues that it has identified using its adverse event reporting system; FDA identifies those potential safety issues from among the tracked safety issues in DARRTS.[24]

Another important aspect of FDA's postmarket safety oversight is monitoring the progress of postmarket studies—conducted after a drug has been approved—that FDA can request or require. Under certain circumstances, FDA can require sponsors to conduct a postmarket study as a condition of approval, such as for drugs granted accelerated approval.[25] The results of postmarket studies provide further information about a drug's safety, efficacy, or optimal use that FDA can use to take one or more actions, such as approving a drug for new uses. Under the accelerated approval program, if sponsors do not conduct the required postmarket study, called a confirmatory trial, with due diligence, or the results of the trial do not confirm the drug's clinical benefit, FDA has the authority to begin procedures for withdrawing the drug's approval for marketing. For example, in 2012, FDA withdrew approval for the NDA for the cancer drug Iressa after the results of its confirmatory trial failed to show an improvement in survival for patients who took it compared with patients who received a placebo. FDA tracks information about postmarket studies, such as their status and projected completion date, in DARRTS.[26] FDA is required to publish an annual report in the Federal Register on the status of certain postmarket studies.[27] In its past reports, FDA has summarized the number of postmarket studies and the extent to which they were proceeding according to established time frames for completion.

Although FDA is responsible for overseeing postmarket studies and ensuring they are completed in a timely manner, we and others have found that, in the past, FDA has not adequately done so. HHS's Office of Inspector General concluded in a 2006 report that FDA could not readily identify whether or how timely postmarket study commitments were progressing toward completion.[28] In 2009, we found that FDA had not been routinely monitoring the status of postmarket studies, primarily because oversight of these studies was not considered a priority.[29] Both reports note that FDA's inadequate oversight was due, in part, to staff not meeting timeliness goals for the review of submissions from sponsors, such as annual status reports that contain information on the progress of postmarket studies and final reports that include results of completed studies. In 2008, FDA hired a contractor to help meet requirements under the Food and Drug Administration Amendments Act of 2007 (FDAAA) that FDA annually review and report on the "backlog" of postmarket studies, which FDA defined as studies that were open (i.e., not fulfilled or released) as of the date of enactment of FDAAA (September 27, 2007).[30] The contractor found that this backlog contained more than 500 postmarket studies where a final report had been submitted that FDA had not yet reviewed, including reports for confirmatory trials that were required for drugs granted accelerated approval.

FDA Granted More than Half of Requests for Fast Track Designation and Denied Most Requests for Breakthrough Therapy Designation

FDA Granted Two-Thirds of Requests for Fast Track Designation and Denied Most Requests for Breakthrough Therapy Designation

Of the 772 requests for fast track designation FDA received from October 1, 2006, through December 31, 2014, FDA granted about two-thirds (or 525) of them. By receiving fast track designation, sponsors may have increased communication with and guidance from FDA officials and may have a rolling review of their drug application. FDA denied about one-fourth (or 207) of the requests for fast track designation; according to FDA officials, requests are generally denied because the drug application does not meet the criteria for fast track designation. For example, requests for fast track designation in which the drug is not intended to treat a serious medical condition will be denied. The 40 remaining requests were either withdrawn by the sponsor or categorized as other by FDA.[31] Since fiscal year 2011, the number of requests FDA has granted fast track designation has increased, from 54 requests granted in fiscal year 2011, to 89 granted in fiscal year 2014. (See figure 1)

In contrast to granting most of the requests for fast track designation, FDA denied more than half (or 120) of the 225 requests for breakthrough therapy designation that the agency received since that expedited program was established in July 2012 through the end of December 2014. According to FDA officials, most requests for this designation are denied because of poor study design associated with the request. FDA granted 71 requests for breakthrough therapy designation since the program was established, including 31 requests granted in each of fiscal years 2013 and 2014. (See figure 2.) According to FDA data, 34 requests for breakthrough therapy designation were withdrawn by the sponsor during the period.

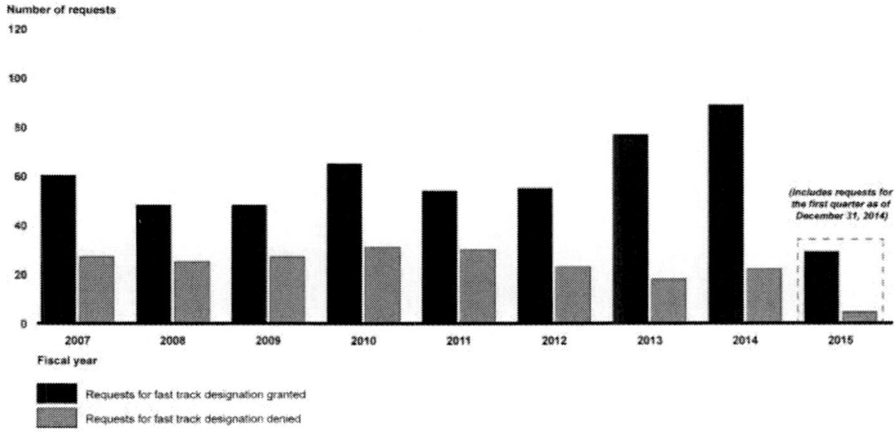

Source: GAO analysis of FDA data. | GAO-16-192.

Notes: In addition to requests granted and denied during the period, 33 requests for fast track designation were withdrawn by the sponsor and 7 were classified by FDA as other. According to FDA, the category of other includes cases where the drug application was inactivated, terminated, or cancelled before FDA made a decision (grant or deny) or if the request is still pending.

Figure 1. Requests the Food and Drug Administration (FDA) Granted and Denied for Fast Track Designation, October 2006 through December 2014.

Antiviral and Oncology Drugs Were the Most Common Product Categories among Applications Granted Fast Track and Breakthrough Therapy Designation

Of the 525 requests for fast track designation that FDA granted from fiscal year 2007 through the first quarter of fiscal year 2015, the most common product category (with 112 requests granted) was for antiviral drugs. For example, Isentress—an antiviral drug to treat human immunodeficiency virus that was approved by FDA in 2007—used fast track designation. This product category was followed by oncology (81 requests granted), neurology (74 requests granted), anti-infectives (55 requests granted), gastroenterology and inborn errors (46 request granted), hematology (34 requests granted), and cardiovascular and renal (32 requests granted). The remaining requests that FDA granted for fast track designation (91 requests) were for drugs in other product categories.32 (See Figure 3.) Appendix I has more information on requests for fast track designation that FDA granted, by product category.

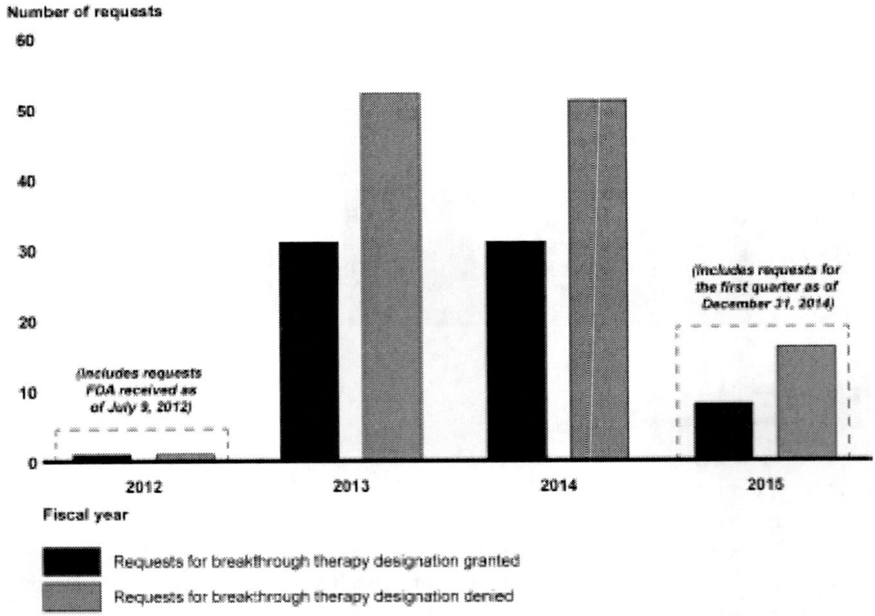

Source: GAO analysis of FDA data. | GAO-16-192.

Notes: The breakthrough therapy designation program was established on July 9, 2012. In addition to requests granted and denied, from July 9, 2012, through December 31, 2014, 34 requests were withdrawn by the sponsor.

Figure 2. Requests the Food and Drug Administration (FDA) Granted and Denied for Breakthrough Therapy Designation, July 9, 2012, through December 31, 2014.

The most common product categories among the 71 requests for which FDA granted breakthrough therapy designation from July 9, 2012, through December 31, 2014, were oncology (15 requests granted), antiviral (14 requests granted), and hematology (14 requests granted).

For example, FDA granted breakthrough therapy designation for the oncology drug Keytruda (a drug to treat patients with advanced melanoma who are no longer responding to other drugs) because, according to FDA, the sponsor demonstrated through preliminary clinical evidence that the drug may offer a substantial improvement over other therapies. The rest of the requests for breakthrough therapy designation FDA granted were for drugs in the FDA product categories of pulmonology, allergy, and rheumatology (7 requests granted); gastroenterology and inborn errors (5 requests granted); psychiatry (4 requests granted), and other (12 requests granted).[33] (See figure 4.)

Appendix II has more information on requests for breakthrough designation that FDA granted, by product category.

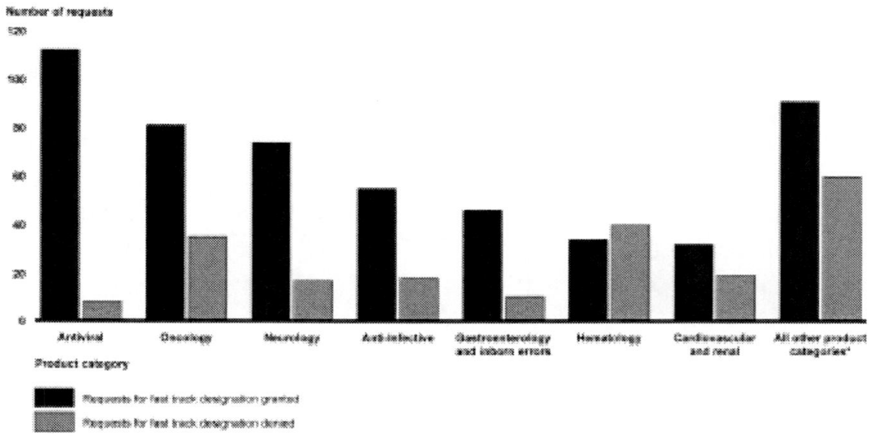

Source: GAO analysis of FDA data. | GAO-16-192.

Notes: In addition to requests granted and denied during the period, 33 requests for fast track designation were withdrawn by the sponsor and 7 requests were classified by FDA as other. According to FDA, the category of other includes cases where the drug application was inactivated, terminated, or cancelled before FDA made a decision (grant or deny) or if the request is still pending.

[a] All other product categories includes the following: anesthesia, analgesia, and addiction; bone, reproductive, and urologic; dermatology and dental; medical imaging; metabolism and endocrinology; psychiatry; pulmonary, allergy, and rheumatology; and transplant and ophthalmology. Each of these product categories had fewer than 5 percent of the total fast track designations granted.

Figure 3. Requests for Fast Track Designation That the Food and Drug Administration (FDA) Granted and Denied, by Product Category, October 2006 through December 2014.

One in Four Drug Applications Approved by FDA Used at Least One Expedited Program, and the Most Frequent Category Was Oncology Drugs

About a quarter of the 1,717 drug applications that FDA approved from October 1, 2006, through December 31, 2014, used at least one expedited program.[34] Drug applications may use multiple expedited programs, although most used one program. Of 444 approved drug applications that used one or more expedited programs, 344 (77 percent) used one expedited program, 78 used 2 programs, 20 used 3 programs, and 2 used all four programs.[35] (See figure 5.) Priority review was the most used program, with 408 of the 444 drug applications (92 percent) receiving priority review. (See figure 6.) Average FDA review time for marketing applications for drugs that used at least one expedited program was less than for drugs that did not. FDA review time was an average of 8.6 months for marketing applications for drugs that used at least one expedited program compared with 12.1 months for marketing applications for drugs that did not.[36]

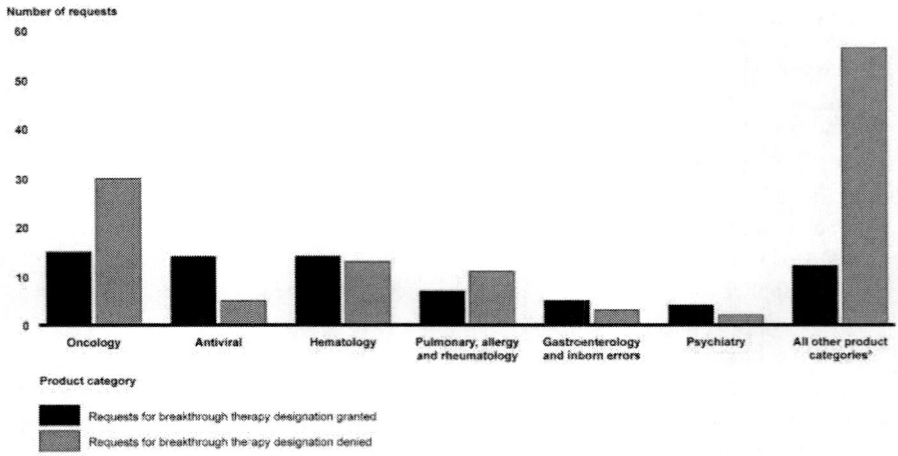

Source: GAO analysis of FDA data. | GAO-16-192.

Notes: The breakthrough therapy designation program was established on July 9, 2012. In addition to requests granted and denied, from July 9, 2012, through December 31, 2014, 34 requests were withdrawn by the sponsor.

[a] All other product categories includes the following: anesthesia, analgesia, and addiction; antiinfectives; cardiovascular and renal; dermatology and dental; neurology; and transplant and ophthalmology. Each of these product categories had fewer than 5 percent of the total breakthrough therapy designations granted.

Figure 4. Requests for Breakthrough Therapy Designation That the Food and Drug Administration (FDA) Granted and Denied, by Product Category, July 9, 2012, through December 31, 2014.

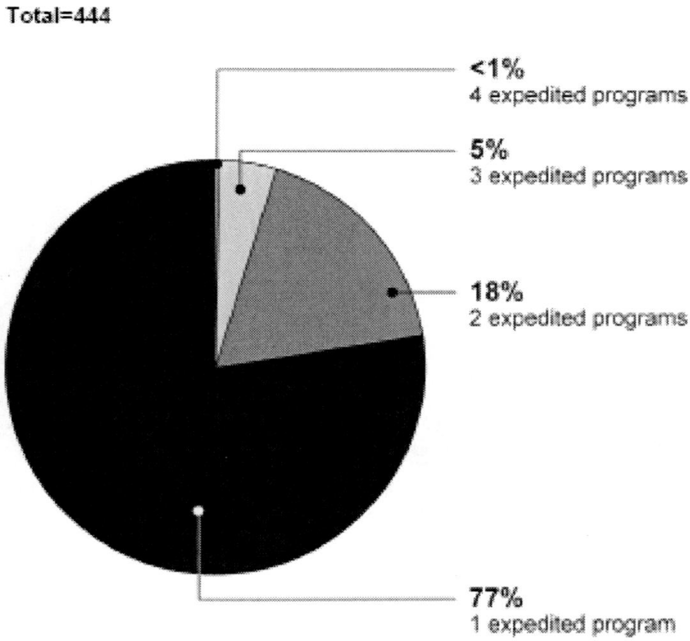

Source: GAO analysis of FDA data. | GAO-16-192.

Note: FDA's Center for Drug Evaluation and Research approved a total of 1,717 new drug applications, biologic license applications, and efficacy supplements during the period, 444 of which used at least one expedited program. Percentages do not add to 100 due to rounding.

Figure 5. Drug Applications Approved by the Food and Drug Administration (FDA) That Used at Least One Expedited Program, Categorized by Number of Expedited Programs, October 2006 through December 2014.

New molecular entities (NME) accounted for 216 (32 percent) of the 685 NDAs that were approved during the time frame of our review.[37] NMEs were more likely to have used an expedited program than NDAs that FDA did not designate as NMEs. Of 216 approved applications for NMEs, FDA data identified 110 (51 percent) of them as using at least one expedited program while 59 of the 469 NDAs that were not NMEs (13 percent) used at least one expedited program.[38] (See figure 7.)

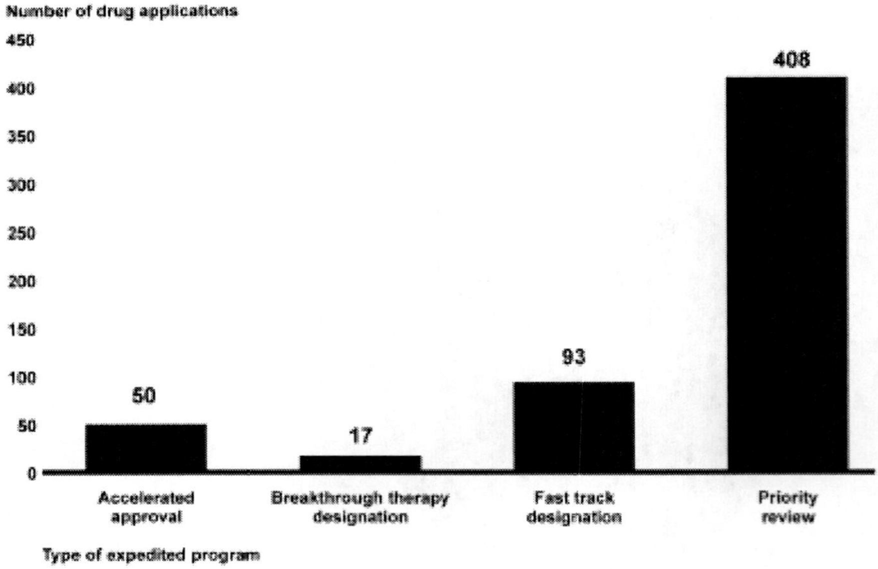

Source: GAO analysis of FDA data. | GAO-16-192.

Notes: Includes new drug applications, biologic license applications, and efficacy supplements that were approved by the Center for Drug Evaluation and Research. Does not sum to total number of approved applications that used an expedited program (444) because applications may use more than one expedited program. The number of approved applications that used the fast track designation may be understated, because, according to FDA officials, prior to November 2013, flagging an application as having used the fast track designation in FDA's database was optional. FDA added a prompt for reviewers to enter whether a drug application used the fast track designation on November 29, 2013.

Figure 6. Number of Drug Applications Approved by the Food and Drug Administration (FDA) That Used an Expedited Program, October 2006 through December 2014.

The most common product category for drug applications approved by FDA from October 1, 2006, through December 31, 2014, that used at least one expedited program was oncology (83 of 444 applications, 19 percent), followed by antiviral (77 applications, 17 percent), and hematology (55 applications, 12 percent). The remaining applications were for drugs in other product categories.[39] (See figure 8.)

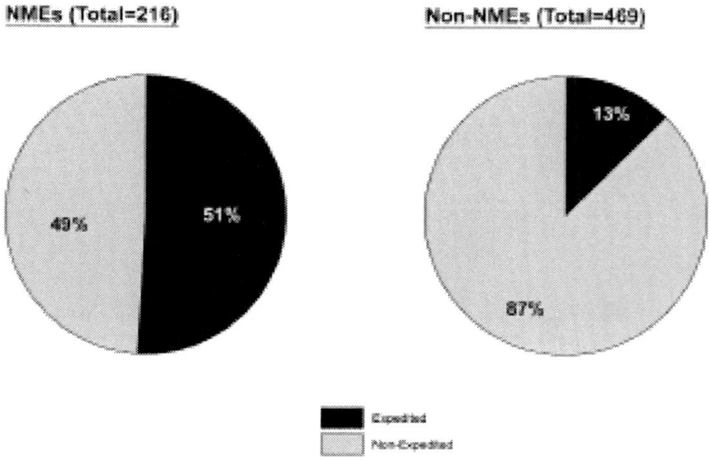

Source: GAO analysis of FDA data. | GAO-16-192.

Note: Analysis includes NDAs approved by FDA's Center for Drug Evaluation and Research. FDA identified approved NDAs as NMEs or non-NMEs in the data we reviewed. FDA does not categorize efficacy supplements or biologic license applications as NMEs.

Figure 7. Comparison of New Drug Applications (NDA) for New Molecular Entities (NME) and Non-NMEs, October 2006 through December 2014.

FDA Lacks Reliable Information for Postmarket Safety Reporting and Oversight

FDA lacks reliable, readily accessible data on tracked safety issues and postmarket studies needed to meet certain postmarket safety reporting responsibilities and to conduct systematic oversight. CDER's internal evaluations of data in its DARRTS database revealed problems with the completeness, timeliness, and accuracy of the data. These problems, as well as problems with the way data are recorded that impair their accessibility, have prevented FDA from publishing some required postmarket safety reports in a timely manner, and have restricted its ability to perform systematic oversight. Internal control standards for the federal government specify that information should be recorded in a form and within a time frame that enables staff to carry out their responsibilities and that relevant, reliable, and timely information should be available for external reporting purposes.[40] Although FDA has taken some steps to address the problems with its data, it lacks comprehensive plans for doing so.

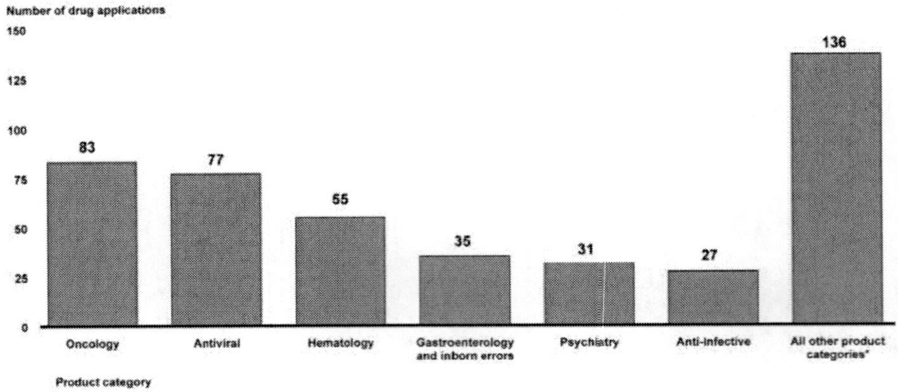

Source: GAO analysis of FDA data. | GAO-16-192.

[a] The other product categories each represented 5 percent or less of all applications that were approved using an expedited program. These other categories were anesthesia, analgesia, and addiction; bone, reproductive, and urologic; cardiovascular and renal; dermatology and dental; medical imaging; metabolism and endocrinology; neurology; pulmonary, allergy, and rheumatology; and transplant and ophthalmology.

Figure 8. Number of Drug Applications Approved by the Food and Drug Administration (FDA) That Used at Least One Expedited Program by Product Category, October 2006 through December 2014.

CDER conducted internal evaluations of its data for tracked safety issues and postmarket studies and found problems with their completeness, timeliness, and accuracy.[41] In addition, our review found that certain information was not readily accessible to FDA staff for analysis.

- *Data on tracked safety issues were incomplete.* CDER's evaluation indicated that the majority of potential safety issues that staff had identified were not being tracked in DARRTS, CDER also identified 144 issues that had not been formally tracked in DARRTS, despite likely meeting CDER's critereia for tracked safety issues.[42] CDER's evaluation indicated that a possible reason that staff were not entering tracked safety issues into DARRTS was due to the time-consuming nature of data entry and the additional requirements associated with conducting a structured, multidisciplinary review, which staff considered burdensome, especially for more straightforward issues. CDER's evaluation compared the entry of tracked safety issues before and after a change in policy that required additional work and found that staff entered roughly two-thirds fewer new tracked safety issues into DARRTS after the new policy went into effect as compared with the year prior. FDA officials we spoke with acknowledged that staff were not following CDER's policies and procedures for tracking and documenting potential safety issues, but said that given the high workload of its review staff it had prioritized identifying, assessing, and addressing potential safety issues over administrative tracking.

- *Postmarket study data were outdated and contained inaccuracies.* CDER's evaluation showed that information on postmarket study status (e.g., whether the study was proceeding according to schedule or was delayed) was often outdated or otherwise inaccurate, partly due to delays in staff reviewing submissions, such as final study reports, from drug sponsors. For example, the evaluation found that over half of reviews of sponsors' submissions associated with about 1,400 postmarket studies FDA requested or required from March 2008 to September 2013 were delayed or overdue.[43] CDER's evaluation also found inaccuracies in the postmarket study data, such as statuses recorded as pending or ongoing that should have been recorded as delayed, as well as delays in data entry. Over a third (500) of the approximately 1,400 studies had their status updated or corrected during the course of CDER's internal evaluation.[44] CDER's evaluation indicated that this pattern of results was similar to the findings of the contractor the agency hired in 2008 to review the backlog of postmarket studies.[45] CDER's internal evaluation of its postmarket study data attributed the data reliability problems to weaknesses in its process that provided numerous opportunities for failures, such as the need to enter data by hand, which could introduce human error, rather than having them automatically populated; lack of automatic linkage between applications and related sponsor submissions, which make them harder to locate; and limited oversight of core steps in the process.

FDA officials we spoke with also indicated that staffing limitations and competing priorities contributed to problems identified with the postmarket study data.[46]

- *Tracked safety issue and postmarket study data were not readily accessible to staff for analysis.* FDA officials told us that DARRTS cannot be queried to determine characteristics of tracked safety issues, such as the therapeutic area of the drug associated with a safety issue, the population affected, or what regulatory actions, if any, FDA took in response to a tracked safety issue. Officials said that such information is contained in the text of electronic documents and must be manually reviewed. Similarly, FDA officials told us that some information about postmarket studies, such as the date FDA requested or required a study, must be manually collected from the text of letters to sponsors; these letters are not automatically linked to information about the study in DARRTS, which can make them challenging to locate.[47]

FDA's lack of reliable, readily accessible postmarket safety data has prevented the agency from publishing required reports in a timely manner and has restricted its ability to conduct systematic oversight.

- *Lack of complete, timely, and accurate data has resulted in FDA not publishing required reports in a timely manner.* As of October 2015, FDA had not published required quarterly reports on potential safety issues identified through its adverse event reporting system for calendar year 2015; FDA officials said they had delayed the report covering January through March 2015 due to ongoing efforts to evaluate the data on tracked safety issues.[48] CDER's internal evaluation found that the number of tracked safety issues included in quarterly reports during the time frame of its review showed a steep decline that did not accurately reflect the agency's actual efforts to identify and evaluate safety issues. In addition, as of October 2015, FDA had not published required annual reports containing data on postmarket studies for fiscal years 2013 and 2014.[49] FDA officials told us that they had decided to delay publication of the reports primarily due to CDER's internal evaluation of the postmarket study data and subsequent efforts to address the data problems that were identified.[50]
- *Lack of reliable and accessible data restricts FDA's ability to conduct systematic oversight of postmarket safety.* CDER's evaluation of tracked safety issues found that when issues were not centrally tracked in DARRTS, they were generally visible only to staff within the division or office that had identified them, which prevented senior management from using DARRTS to systematically determine whether safety issues were being evaluated and actions were being

taken within reasonable time frames. FDA officials subsequently told us that they have other mechanisms for informing management about potential safety issues outside of DARRTS, such as including them in weekly reports that are discussed at senior management team meetings; however, none of these mechanisms is comprehensive of all potential safety issues CDER staff are evaluating. FDA officials also told us that they cannot readily conduct certain analyses, such as how often and what type of actions FDA has taken for drugs by therapeutic area (e.g., oncology or psychiatry drugs). Similarly, problems with FDA's postmarket study data limit FDA's ability to conduct certain analyses. Inability to quickly determine when postmarket studies were established, for example, does not allow agency staff to readily construct cohorts of studies requested or required in a given fiscal year, which would be necessary for FDA to conduct analyses on completion rates over time, or to review information on studies that were requested or required before and after certain legislative or policy changes to examine their effect.

FDA has reported taking steps to address the problems it identified with the postmarket safety data in DARRTS, but the agency does not have comprehensive plans with goals and time frames.

- *FDA intends to address its incomplete data on tracked safety issues by revising and streamlining its processes for reviewing and tracking these issues*. FDA officials said that CDER has formed a workgroup that is considering options to clarify which potential safety issues should be centrally tracked, and how the tracking and review processes could be streamlined. Officials did not provide an estimate for when these processes would be revised. In the meantime, the Office of New Drugs within CDER issued an interim set of guidelines for staff in April 2015 that state that all potential safety issues requiring further evaluation must be entered into DARRTS. The guidelines also instruct staff to retroactively enter tracked safety issues into DARRTS to enhance the completeness of the data.[51] According to FDA officials, these guidelines are an interim measure to provide key information to staff while CDER's processes for reviewing and tracking safety issues are being revised.
- *FDA intends to increase the timeliness and accuracy of its postmarket study data by improving tools for oversight and data collection*. FDA

officials said the agency is aiming to facilitate more timely review of sponsor submissions that contain information on postmarket studies by improving internal oversight. In the fall of 2014, FDA implemented new reporting capabilities that provide information to the review divisions within CDER on a monthly basis about all open postmarket studies those divisions oversee, such as annual status reports and final reports received from sponsors and what the goal dates are for their review. Officials said they have also begun meeting with the Office of Business Informatics within CDER to discuss improvements that could be made in FDA's new information technology platform, such as automated collection of certain types of data. FDA officials told us that the new platform will include the date.

FDA requested or required a postmarket study in a form that can be queried.[52]

- *FDA lacks comprehensive plans to address the problems with its tracked safety issue and postmarket study data.* FDA officials told us that, while the agency has multiple efforts under way to improve its tracked safety issue and postmarket study data, it has not developed plans that comprehensively outline these efforts, establish related goals, and provide time frames for their completion. Additionally, FDA officials said they do not have plans to analyze tracked safety issue and postmarket study data to inform the agency's oversight of its expedited programs, such as determining if drugs that used an expedited program were subsequently associated with tracked safety issues at rates or of types that differed from drugs that used FDA's standard process. FDA officials said that they do not subject applications that used an expedited program to greater postmarket safety monitoring and they do not have plans to do so because, to obtain approval for marketing, these applications are required to meet the same standard of evidence for safety and effectiveness as are applications that used FDA's standard process.[53] However, some of the expedited programs specifically permit the use of fewer, shorter, or smaller clinical trials during development, and FDA's lack of analysis means that the agency lacks comprehensive information on whether drugs that were developed under these programs pose additional safety risks to patients once they are available on the market.

CONCLUSION

Complete, accurate, and timely postmarket safety data, such as information on tracked safety issues and the progress of postmarket studies, are essential for FDA to meet its responsibility to monitor the safety of marketed drugs. FDA's monitoring efforts once drugs reach the market are particularly important for those drugs that have used certain expedited programs to reduce the development time before approval, where there may be greater potential for previously unrecognized safety issues to appear once a drug is more widely used. FDA has supported efforts to shorten development and streamline the agency's review of drug applications through expedited pathways. However, we found problems with the agency's efforts to oversee and track potential safety issues and postmarket studies once those drugs are on the market. While internal control standards for the federal government specify that information should be recorded in a form and within a time frame that enables staff to carry out their responsibilities and that relevant, reliable, and timely information should be available for external reporting purposes, FDA's data on postmarket safety issues and studies were found to be incomplete, outdated, to contain inaccuracies, and to be stored in a manner that made routine, systematic analysis difficult.

To effectively track potential safety issues and the agency's response to them, and to track and ensure postmarket studies are being conducted on schedule, it is important that FDA have ready access to complete, timely, and accurate information. This information also provides the basis for FDA's required reports, which are important for informing policymakers and the public about emerging safety issues and the extent to which drug sponsors are fulfilling their obligations to conduct studies on the safety, efficacy, and optimal use of marketed drugs. Reliable and accessible data would also provide FDA with information to conduct analyses to inform oversight of its expedited programs. Although FDA officials have pointed out that all applications have to meet the same statutory standards for approval, and that additional risks posed by applications that used an expedited program may be acceptable given the seriousness of conditions being treated, we believe that reliable data to support additional oversight is important given public concern about the safety implications of streamlined drug development and review. While FDA has begun some efforts to improve its data by issuing guidelines for staff and adding tools for oversight, more concrete plans to correct known problems with the completeness, timeliness, and accuracy of its data, and to improve underlying data systems so that information important for oversight is captured in a useable form, are critical.

RECOMMENDATIONS FOR EXECUTIVE ACTION

To improve the data on tracked safety issues and postmarket studies that are needed for required reporting and for systematic oversight of postmarket drug safety, we recommend that the Secretary of HHS direct the Commissioner of FDA to take the following two actions:

- develop comprehensive plans, with goals and time frames, to help ensure that identified problems with the completeness, timeliness, and accuracy of information in its database on tracked safety issues and postmarket studies are corrected, and
- work with stakeholders within FDA to identify additional improvements that could be made to FDA's current database or future information technology investments to capture information in a form that can be easily and systematically used by staff for oversight purposes.

AGENCY COMMENTS AND OUR EVALUATION

We provided a draft of this report to HHS for comment. In its written comments, HHS concurred with our recommendations and stated that conducting rigorous oversight of postmarket safety is a priority. HHS noted that FDA, by improving its data on postmarket studies and tracked safety issues, can more effectively use these data to monitor drugs in the postmarket setting. HHS also provided technical comments that we incorporated, as appropriate.

In addition, HHS commented that drugs using an expedited program must meet the same statutory standards for safety and effectiveness to be approved for the U.S. market as other, non-expedited drugs—a point that is included in our report. HHS noted that drugs using the accelerated approval program are also required to complete postmarket studies for the drug sponsors to verify the anticipated clinical benefits. We believe that this reliance on postapproval studies for verification of the clinical benefits of drugs entering the U.S.

market using accelerated approval underscores the importance of improved FDA oversight of postmarket studies. HHS also pointed out the differences between the standards for granting breakthrough therapy designation or fast track designation—that is, the ability for a drug sponsor to use one of these two expedited programs—and FDA approval of the drugs for marketing; these distinctions are also noted in our report.

HHS also commented that FDA-approved drugs that used an expedited program do not necessarily require different postmarket safety monitoring than other drugs, noting that tracked safety issues and postmarket studies are utilized to monitor all drugs after they are approved by FDA, including drugs using an expedited program. However, as we note in our report, some of the expedited programs specifically permit the use of fewer, shorter, or smaller clinical trials during development, and FDA has noted that additional risks posed by applications that use an expedited program may be acceptable given the seriousness of conditions being treated. FDA's lack of analysis of data on tracked safety issues and postmarket studies related to applications that used an expedited program indicates that the agency lacks comprehensive information on whether drugs that were developed under these programs pose additional safety risks to patients once they are available on the market. We believe that maintaining reliable data that could be used to conduct such analysis is critical, given public concern about the safety implications of streamlined drug development and review.

HHS acknowledged the challenges of FDA's administrative tracking of postmarket safety issues and commented that CDER's internal evaluations, which CDER initiated before we started our review, had helped identify these challenges. HHS further noted that FDA is taking steps to address some of these challenges related to its internal data. HHS also listed other mechanisms FDA uses to monitor postmarket safety issues and the status of its "backlog" of postmarket studies, noting that CDER staff prioritized identifying, evaluating, communicating about, and taking regulatory action to address safety issues over expending limited resources on entering information about safety issues into FDA's tracking system. Nonetheless, given that FDA's internal evaluations found that information on postmarket studies was often outdated or otherwise inaccurate, we continue to believe that complete, accurate, and timely data are necessary for FDA managers to have the information required to conduct systematic oversight and appropriately monitor tracked safety issues and postmarket studies.

Sincerely yours,

Marcia Crosse,
Director, Health Care

APPENDIX I: NUMBER OF GRANTED REQUESTS FOR FAST TRACK DESIGNATION BY PRODUCT CATEGORY, FISCAL YEARS 2007 THROUGH 2015

	Number granted fast track designation by the Food and Drug Administration's (FDA) Center for Drug Evaluation and Research, by fiscal year										
Product category	2007	2008	2009	2010	2011	2012	2013	2014	2015[a]	2007 2015[a]	%
Antiviral	13	9	11	23	20	8	13	12	3	112	21.3
Oncology	14	4	7	9	10	9	8	18	2	81	15.4
Neurology	6	11	9	8	8	6	8	14	4	74	14.1
Anti-infective	5	3	2	4	1	4	15	15	6	55	10.5
Gastroenterology and inborn errors	6	2	6	4	6	6	6	6	4	46	8.8
Hematology	3	1	2	4	3	6	5	8	2	34	6.5
Cardiovascular and renal	7	4	5	2	1	4	3	5	1	32	6.1
Anesthesia, analgesia, and addiction	0	4	0	3	2	3	4	7	0	23	4.4
Transplant and ophthalmology	3	2	2	3	1	2	1	0	5	19	3.6
Pulmonary, allergy, and rheumatology	2	4	3	2	2	1	2	0	1	17	3.2
Psychiatry	0	1	1	1	0	5	6	2	0	16	3.1
Medical imaging	0	2	0	1	0	0	2	1	0	6	1.1
Bone, reproductive, and urologic	0	1	0	1	0	0	2	0	1	5	1.0
Dermatology and dental	1	0	0	0	0	1	1	1	0	4	0.8
Metabolism and endocrinology	0	0	0	0	0	0	1	0	0	1	0.2
Total	60	48	48	65	54	55	77	89	29	525	100.0

Source: GAO analysis of FDA data. | GAO-16-192.

Notes: FDA product categories generally correspond to the FDA review division.

[a]Data for fiscal year 2015 include requests through the first quarter (as of December 31, 2014).

Appendix II: Number of Granted Requests for Breakthrough Therapy Designation by Product Category, July 9, 2012, through December 31, 2014

	Number granted breakthrough therapy designation by the Food and Drug Administration's (FDA) Center for Drug Evaluation and Research, by fiscal year					
Product category	2012[a]	2013	2014	2015[b]	2012-2015[a,b]	%
Oncology	0	6	7	2	15	21.1
Antiviral	0	8	5	1	14	19.7
Hematology	0	7	7	0	14	19.7
Pulmonary, allergy, and rheumatology	1	1	3	2	7	9.9
Gastroenterology and inborn errors	0	3	1	1	5	7.0
Psychiatry	0	1	2	1	4	5.6
Neurology	0	3	0	0	3	4.2
Anesthesia, analgesia, and addiction	0	0	2	0	2	2.8
Anti-infective	0	0	2	0	2	2.8
Dermatology and dental	0	1	1	0	2	2.8
Transplant and ophthalmology	0	0	1	1	2	2.8
Cardiovascular and renal	0	1	0	0	1	1.4
Total	1	31	31	8	71	100.0

Source: GAO analysis of FDA data. | GAO-16-192.

Notes: Breakthrough therapy designation was established under the Food and Drug Administration Safety and Innovation Act, enacted on July 9, 2012. FDA product categories generally correspond to the FDA review division.

Percentage rows do not sum to 100 due to rounding.

[a] Data for fiscal year 2012 include requests FDA received as of July 9, 2012.

[b] Data for fiscal year 2015 include requests through the first quarter (as of December 31, 2014).

End Notes

[1] Within FDA, the Center for Drug Evaluation and Research is responsible for overseeing the safety and effectiveness of drugs sold in the United States.

[2] Janet Woodcock, M.D., Director, Center for Drug Evaluation and Research, FDA, 21st Century Cures: Modernizing Clinical Trials and Incorporating the Patient Perspective – Dr. Woodcock, testimony before the House Subcommittee on Health, Committee on Energy and Commerce, 113th Cong., 2nd sess., July 11, 2014.

[3] See, for example, Jonathan J. Darrow, et al., "New FDA Breakthrough-Drug Category – Implications for Patients," New England Journal of Medicine, vol. 370, no. 13 (2014) and T.J. Moore and C.D. Furberg, "The Safety Risks of Innovation: The FDA's Expedited Drug Development Pathway," Journal of the American Medical Association, vol. 308, no. 9 (2012).

[4] 21 U.S.C. §§ 355(k)(5)(A), 356b(c).

[5] For this report, we use the term postmarket studies to refer to the studies and trials that FDA requires drug sponsors to conduct (known as postmarketing requirements) and those that FDA requests and drug sponsors agree to conduct (known as postmarketing commitments). FDA is required by law to publish reports on certain potential safety issues and postmarket studies; these reports help to inform external stakeholders about emerging safety issues and the agency's response to them, and whether drug sponsors are completing postmarket studies according to established time frames. 21 U.S.C. §§ 355(k), 356b(c).

[6] See, for example, GAO, Drug Safety: Improvement Needed in FDA's Postmarket Decision-making and Oversight Process, GAO-06-402 (Washington, D.C.: Mar. 31, 2006); A. Baciu, K. Stratton, and S. P. Burke, eds., Institute of Medicine of the National Academies, Committee on the Assessment of the U.S. Drug Safety System, The Future of Drug Safety: Promoting and Protecting the Health of the Public (Washington, D.C.: Sept. 22, 2006); and GAO, Drug Safety: FDA Has Begun Efforts to Enhance Postmarket Safety, but Additional Actions Are Needed, GAO-10-68 (Washington, D.C.: Nov. 9, 2009).

[7] For example, see Bo Wang and Aaron S. Kesselheim, "Characteristics of Efficacy Evidence Supporting Approval of Supplemental Indications for Prescription Drugs in United States, 2005–14: Systematic Review," British Medical Journal (2015), and Chul Kim and Vinay Prasad, "Cancer Drugs Approved on the Basis of a Surrogate End Point and Subsequent Overall Survival: An Analysis of 5 Years of U.S. Food and Drug Administration Approvals," Journal of the American Medical Association Internal Medicine (2015), accessed October 27, 2015, http://archinte.jamanetwork.com/article.aspx?Articleid=2463590.

[8] We also issued a separate report describing postmarket studies for medical devices. See GAO, Medical Devices: FDA Ordered Postmarket Studies to Better Understand Safety Issues, and Many Studies Are Ongoing, GAO-15-815 (Washington, D.C.: Sept. 30, 2015).

[9] As previously mentioned, irrespective of their use of expedited programs, sponsors are required to submit a marketing application to FDA before a drug can be approved for marketing in the United States.

[10] For our analysis, we included all requests for fast track and breakthrough designation, including requests associated with investigational new drug applications and with other drug applications, such as new drug applications. A sponsor must submit an investigational new drug application that summarizes the data that have been collected on the compound and outlines plans for the clinical trials. According to FDA officials, fast track and breakthrough therapy designation may be granted for an investigational new drug or later, such as when a new drug application is submitted. The Food and Drug Administration Safety and Innovation Act, signed into law in 2012, required FDA to establish breakthrough therapy designation. Pub. L. No. 112-144, § 902, 126 Stat. 993, 1086 (2012) (amending the Federal Food, Drug, and Cosmetic Act § 506; codified at 21 U.S.C. § 356).

[11] FDA extracted data from its database for fast track designation in two rounds—fast track data through September 30, 2010, were extracted on May 31, 2015, and fast track data after September 30, 2010, were extracted on June 2, 2015. FDA extracted data for breakthrough therapy designation on April 30, 2015.

[12] Efficacy supplements to NDAs and BLAs are applications to make certain changes (e.g., adding a new indication for use) to an approved marketing application. FDA's Center for Biologics Evaluation and Research also reviews certain BLAs for biologics such as blood products, vaccines, and allergenic products. We did not review BLAs reviewed by the Center for Biologics Evaluation and Research; our review included NDAs, BLAs, and efficacy supplements reviewed by CDER.

[13] The data we analyzed may understate the number of approved applications that used the fast track designation prior to November 2013, because, according to FDA officials, reviewers were not required to record the fast track designation in the FDA database at that time. As a result, although FDA had conducted some manual data checks to update the database, some applications approved from October 2006 through November 2013, that we analyzed may have used the fast track designation but were not flagged as such in the data FDA provided and therefore would not be counted in our analysis. FDA required reviewers to enter whether a drug application used the fast track designation beginning on November 29, 2013.

[14] Tracked safety issues are potential safety issues with marketed drugs that FDA has determined are significant and are tracked in one of its internal databases. We received and reviewed FDA data on tracked safety issues related to drug applications approved by CDER for the same fiscal year 2007 through the first quarter of fiscal year 2015 period. For postmarket studies, we reviewed data FDA had previously compiled for the HHS Office of Inspector General on postmarketing requirements that were related to applications approved by CDER during fiscal years 2008 through 2014. We used these data and discussions with FDA on shortcomings in these data, to inform our evaluation of the extent to which FDA's data were sufficient for FDA to perform its postmarket reporting and oversight responsibilities.

[15] These evaluations were conducted by CDER staff and presented to senior leadership starting in February 2013. We reviewed 5 slide presentations summarizing the results of these evaluations, the latest of which was dated March 2015. According to CDER officials, these slide presentations presented the results of internal evaluations conducted by CDER staff; they do not represent formal FDA findings or conclusions.

[16] See GAO, Standards for Internal Control in the Federal Government, GAO/AIMD-00- 21.3.1 (Washington, D.C.: Nov. 1, 1999). Internal control is synonymous with management control and comprises the plans, methods, and procedures used to meet missions, goals, and objectives.

[17] In its guidance on expedited programs, FDA defines unmet medical needs as conditions whose treatment or diagnosis are not addressed adequately by available treatments. FDA considers drugs to address an unmet medical need when there are no other available treatments, or when the drug improves upon available treatments. See Department of Health and Human Services, Food and Drug Administration, Guidance for Industry: Expedited Programs for Serious Conditions – Drugs and Biologics, (Silver Spring, Md.: May 2014). Drugs may also be reviewed under an expedited program in certain circumstances, such as if a sponsor submits its drug application with a priority review voucher. Priority review vouchers are incentives that are awarded by FDA, for example, after a sponsor develops and receives approval for a drug to treat a rare pediatric disease. The voucher entitles the sponsor to receive priority review for a future drug application of its choosing. As of September 24, 2015, FDA had issued 7 priority review vouchers and had not approved a drug application from a sponsor redeeming a voucher as of December 31, 2014.

[18] For accelerated approval, a surrogate endpoint is a laboratory measure or physical sign that is reasonably likely to predict clinical benefit, but is not itself a measure of clinical benefit. For example, tumor shrinkage in certain cancer types has been considered reasonably likely to predict an improvement in overall survival. Similarly, for this expedited program, an intermediate clinical endpoint is a measurement of a therapeutic effect that can be measured earlier than an effect on irreversible morbidity or mortality and is considered reasonably likely to predict the drug's effect on irreversible morbidity or mortality or other clinical benefit. A clinical endpoint is a direct measure of how a patient feels, functions, or survives.

[19] In addition, studies have shown that total development time (i.e., years between initial FDA approval to begin human testing and approval to market the drug) is shorter for drugs approved through an expedited program. For example, a study that examined development times for novel new drugs approved in 2008, and compared expedited programs (fast track designation, accelerated approval, and priority review) to standard review, reported that total development time was shortened by over 2 years, from a median of 7.5 years to a median of 5.1 years. See T. J. Moore and C. D. Furberg, "Development Times, Clinical Testing, Postmarket Follow-up, and Safety Risks for the New Drugs Approved by the U.S. Food and Drug Administration: The Class of 2008," Journal of the American Medical Association Internal Medicine, vol. 174, no. 1 (2014).

[20] FDA can rescind breakthrough therapy designation or fast track designation if a drug no longer meets the qualifying criteria; for example, if another drug is subsequently approved and the drug application under review no longer addresses an unmet medical need. Additionally, the drug sponsor can also withdraw its request for review using an expedited program.

[21] Department of Health and Human Services, Food and Drug Administration, Guidance for Industry: Expedited Programs for Serious Conditions – Drugs and Biologics, (Silver Spring, Md.: May 2014). Under accelerated approval, a drug application may be approved based on a surrogate or intermediate clinical endpoint with a study to verify the clinical benefit required after the drug is marketed. According to FDA officials, although there is a risk that a drug granted accelerated approval ultimately will not be shown to provide actual clinical benefit, most drugs granted accelerated approval successfully demonstrate clinical benefit.

[22] To obtain approval to market a drug, a sponsor must demonstrate that the drug is safe and provide evidence, based on adequate and well-controlled trials, that the drug is effective for its intended purpose. 21 U.S.C. § 355(d), 21 C.F.R. § 314.126 (2014).

[23] FDA began tracking safety issues in DARRTS in January 2007, in response to a recommendation from our 2006 report, GAO-06-402, and following a report from the Institute of Medicine, The Future of Drug Safety. According to FDA, almost 1,000 tracked safety issues were entered into DARRTS from January 2007 to March 2012.

[24] 21 U.S.C. § 355(k)(5)(A). Specifically, FDA is required by law to publish a quarterly report of any new safety information or potential signal of a serious risk identified through its adverse event reporting system within the last quarter. As a matter of process, CDER identifies those safety signals that meet statutory criteria for quarterly reporting from its tracked safety issues. Tracked safety issues that arise from other sources, such as epidemiologic studies or other published literature, are not included in these quarterly reports.

[25] In addition to studies required as a condition of accelerated approval, FDA can also require sponsors to conduct postmarketing studies (1) to assess a known serious risk, assess signals of serious risk, or identify an unexpected serious risk related to the use of a drug when available data indicate the potential for a serious risk; (2) to study certain drugs for pediatric populations, when these drugs are not adequately labeled for use in pediatric populations; and (3) to demonstrate safety and efficacy in humans for a drug approved on the basis of

animal efficacy data because human trials were not ethical or feasible. FDA may also request a study known as a postmarketing commitment. A postmarketing commitment is a study that sponsor agrees to, but is not required to conduct after drug approval.

[26] The status of a postmarket study is determined by FDA based on information from the sponsor about its progress, and is generally determined based on the original schedule. FDA categorizes postmarket studies as open or closed. Open postmarket studies are classified by FDA as pending (not started but not past the date the sponsor projected the study would start); ongoing (proceeding according to or ahead of the original schedule); delayed (proceeding but behind the sponsor's original schedule); terminated (ended before completion, but the sponsor has yet to submit a final report to FDA); or submitted (ended and the sponsor has submitted a final report FDA). Closed postmarket studies are classified by FDA as fulfilled (FDA has determined that the sponsor has met the terms of the commitment or requirement) or released (the sponsor was no longer obligated to conduct the study because it was considered no longer feasible, because it would no longer provide useful information, or because the product was withdrawn).

[27] 21 U.S.C. § 356b(c).

[28] This report contained recommendations, including that FDA improve its information system for monitoring postmarketing studies so that it provides timely, accurate, and useful information, and that FDA ensure that postmarketing studies are being monitored. FDA agreed with these recommendations. See Department of Health and Human Services, Office of Inspector General, FDA's Monitoring of Postmarketing Study Commitments, OEI-01-04-00390 (Washington, D.C.; June 2006). HHS's Office of Inspector General is currently conducting a study that examines, among other things, how FDA monitors postmarketing requirements.

[29] See GAO, New Drug Approval: FDA Needs to Enhance Its Oversight of Drugs Approved on the Basis of Surrogate Endpoints, GAO-09-866 (Washington, D.C.: Sept. 23, 2009).

[30] Pub. L. No. 110-85, § 921, 121 Stat. 823, 962 (2007) (adding 21 U.S.C. § 355(k)(5)(C)). According to FDA, the contractor found 63 percent of studies in the backlog were initially labeled as pending, whereas at the end of the contractor's review, 14 percent were labeled as pending.

[31] According to FDA, requests for fast track designation with a status of other include cases where the drug application is inactivated, terminated, or cancelled before FDA made a decision to grant or deny the sponsor's request or FDA's decision on the request was still pending at the time FDA extracted the data for our review.

[32] The other product categories for which fast track designation was granted—each of which had fewer than 5 percent of the total fast track designations granted—were anesthesia, analgesia, and addiction (23 requests granted); transplant and ophthalmology (19 requests granted); pulmonary, allergy, and rheumatology (17 requests granted); psychiatry (16 requests granted); medical imaging (6 requests granted); bone, reproductive, and urologic (5 requests granted); dermatology and dental (4 requests granted); and metabolism and endocrinology (1 request granted).

[33] The other product categories for which breakthrough therapy designation was granted— each of which had fewer than 5 percent of the total breakthrough therapy designations granted—were neurology (3 requests granted); anesthesia, analgesia, and addiction (2 requests granted); anti-infectives (2 requests granted); dermatology and dental (2 requests granted); transplant and ophthalmology (2 requests granted); and cardiovascular and renal (1 request granted).

[34] The 1,717 drug applications included in our review were NDAs, BLAs, and efficacy supplements approved by CDER.

[35] The new cancer drugs ibrutinib and nivolumab used all four expedited programs. Ibrutinib was approved in November 2013 for a rare form of blood cancer and works by blocking the action of an enzyme that allows cancer cells to grow and divide. Nivolumab was approved in December 2014 to treat skin cancer and works by helping the body's immune system to attack tumors.

[36] This difference is statistically significant. Results may primarily reflect the effect of priority review, which shortens FDA's goal time for taking action on a marketing application, because most approved applications that used one or more expedited programs received priority review.

[37] FDA classifies certain drugs as NMEs for purposes of its review. Many of these products contain active chemical substances that have not been approved by FDA previously. Our analysis of NMEs excludes BLAs and NDA- and BLA-related efficacy supplements because FDA does not classify these applications as NMEs.

[38] This difference is statistically significant.

[39] These other product categories were anesthesia, analgesia, and addiction; antiinfectives; bone, reproductive, and urologic; cardiovascular and renal; dermatology and dental; gastroenterology and inborn errors; medical imaging; metabolism and endocrinology; neurology; psychiatry; pulmonary, allergy, and rheumatology; and transplant and ophthalmology.

[40] GAO/AIMD-00-21.3.1.

[41] CDER staff performed an evaluation of the tracked safety issue data in DARRTS and presented the results to senior leadership in April 2013, October 2014, and March 2015. CDER's evaluation of postmarket study data in DARRTS was presented to senior leadership in February 2013 and October 2014.

[42] CDER officials noted that this analysis of safety issues that likely met criteria to be formally tracked had several limitations, including that the process to determine whether a given issue should have been entered into DARRTS as a tracked safety issue was subjective, was performed by staff not involved in the identification or assessment of the safety issues, and was based on limited information about the safety issues.

[43] Sponsor submissions comprised annual status reports that provide information on the progress of postmarket studies and final reports that include results of completed studies. We defined "delayed" as reviews of these submissions that had been completed later than they should have been based on CDER's goal time frames and "overdue" as reviews that were late with respect to CDER's goal time frames and were still outstanding at the time of CDER's evaluation. The evaluation examined sponsor submissions associated with NDAs and BLAs reviewed by CDER.

[44] FDA officials told us that the 500 updates were as-reported by review staff based on their recollections. They also explained that CDER's analysis could not determine the specific reasons for the status updates—that is, how many of the 500 status updates occurred because (1) a review was not conducted in a timely manner, (2) there was an error in determining or entering the status into DARRTS, or (3) the sponsor had progressed with the study between the time of the last status update and the time of CDER's internal evaluation and the updated data entry.

[45] See Booz Allen Hamilton, Independent Evaluation of FDA's Prescription Drug User Fee Act – Evaluations and Initiatives; CDER Technical Support and Analysis, Deliverable 2-8: Final Report on the PMR/PMC Backlog Review, April 10, 2009, accessed November 5, 2015,

http://www.fda.gov/downloads/drugs/guidancecomplianceregulatoryinformation/post-marketingphaseivcommitments/ucm181135.pdf, and Booz Allen Hamilton, CDER Analysis, Evaluation and Technical Assistance, Deliverable 6: Final Report on the PMR/PMC Backlog Review, March 12, 2010, accessed October 29, 2015, http://www.fda.gov/downloads/drugs/guidancecomplianceregulatoryinformation/post-marketingphaseivcommitments/ucm232880.pdf. FDA is required to report annually to Congress on the backlog of postmarket studies—which FDA defined as studies that were open (i.e., not fulfilled or released) as of September 27, 2007—and to assign start dates and estimated completion dates for such studies.

[46] FDA officials we spoke with said that CDER does not have enough review staff because of, among other things, staff attrition and difficulties in recruiting staff with specialized skills. Officials estimated that the Office of New Drugs within CDER was approximately 10 percent under its authorized staffing ceiling. They also said that competing priorities, such as the need to review drug applications within time frames established by Prescription Drug User Fee Act, and communicate with external stakeholders, had forced the agency to prioritize its work. For example, although final study reports are expected to be reviewed within 12 months of receipt, officials said that this is an aspirational goal and dependent on resources and staffing capacity.

[47] Officials told us that while they can estimate the date a study was requested or required using a proxy method, this method relies on data that are not always complete or accurate and still requires manual review to correct discrepancies.

[48] As of October 2015, the most recent quarterly report available on FDA's website was for October through December 2014, which FDA posted on July 28, 2015.

[49] As of October 2015, the most recent annual report in the Federal Register was for fiscal year 2012. See Notice of Availability, Report on the Performance of Drug and Biologics Firms in Conducting Postmarketing Requirements and Commitments; Availability, 79 Fed. Reg. 9230 (Feb. 18, 2014).

[50] FDA has also delayed publishing mandated annual reports to Congress on its backlog of postmarket studies (studies that were open (i.e., not fulfilled or released) as of September 27, 2007). FDA submitted reports to Congress covering fiscal years 2012, 2013, and 2014 in November 2015.

[51] Officials said that as of August 2015, 102 tracked safety issues had been retroactively entered into DARRTS. CDER aims to complete retroactive entry of tracked safety issues by March 30, 2016.

[52] FDA is in the process of implementing its new informatics platform, Panorama, and plans to move away from using DARRTS once it is fully in place. Officials told us that they do not expect Panorama to take on postmarket safety functions within the next 3 years and did not provide an estimate of when this would occur. In the meantime, officials said that the Office of Business Informatics has added the capability in DARRTS to record the date studies were requested or required; this information will be entered for all new postmarket studies as of October 1, 2015.

[53] Although FDA has noted that greater risk may be acceptable for drugs that treat life-threatening and severely debilitating diseases, FDA officials also told us that they consider whether or not a drug used an expedited program to be a poor indicator for the need for enhanced postmarket monitoring. For example, officials said it is possible that a postmarket study related to an expedited application might examine a safety issue that affects a small number of patients, whereas a study not related to an expedited application might examine a safety issue with the potential to affect a large number of patients.

In: FDA's Expedited Drug Programs
Editor: Gary Lawrence
ISBN: 978-1-63485-772-7

Chapter 2

STATEMENT OF JANET WOODCOCK, DIRECTOR, CENTER FOR DRUG EVALUATION AND RESEARCH, FOOD AND DRUG ADMINISTRATION. HEARING ON "21ST CENTURY CURES: INCORPORATING THE PATIENT PERSPECTIVE"*

INTRODUCTION

Mr. Chairman, Ranking Member Pallone, and Members of the Subcommittee, I am Dr. Janet Woodcock, Director of the Center for Drug Evaluation and Research (CDER) at the Food and Drug Administration (FDA or the Agency), which is part of the Department of Health and Human Services (HHS). Thank you for the opportunity to be here today to discuss modernizing clinical trials, incorporating the patient perspective, and several FDA activities intended to promote pharmaceutical innovation.

In recent years, there have been important advances to help ensure that therapies for serious conditions are approved and available to patients as soon as there are sufficient data to show that the therapies' benefits outweigh their risks. Despite this progress, there is much more work to be done. Many scientific discoveries still need to be translated into treatments for patients in need of new lifesaving therapies.

---

* This is an edited, reformatted and augmented version of a statement presented July 11, 2014 before the House Committee on Energy and Commerce, Subcommittee on Health.

FDA is committed to doing our part to help bridge this gap. We have been actively scrutinizing, strengthening, and streamlining our regulatory processes at various steps along the path from drug discovery to drug approval, including the clinical development phase—the longest and most expensive period of drug development. As part of this effort, we have developed and successfully used a number of flexible and innovative approaches to expedite the development and review of drugs to the benefit of millions of Americans. FDA routinely works closely with drug sponsors to apply flexibility, including use of biomarkers, surrogate endpoints, nontraditional trial designs, and other available tools to expedite the development of products to treat both common and rare diseases. Particularly for drugs intended to treat life-threatening and severely debilitating illnesses, FDA exercises the broadest flexibility in applying its statutory standards. We also have initiated and participated in many efforts to address the underlying scientific and clinical trial infrastructure challenges that affect the cost and timeliness of drug development. Some of these challenges need to be addressed by those outside of FDA; but we continue to look for ways to streamline the clinical development phase, where possible and within our purview.

Statement of the Problem

FDA's approval process is now faster than anywhere else in the world. Just last year, three-quarters of the new drugs FDA approved were approved in the United States before the European Union (EU) and Japan. Currently 90 percent of drugs that represent an advance over existing treatment are reviewed and decided on in 180 days, some in considerably fewer days.

Despite the growing success and speed of the approval process and revolutionary advances in genomics more than a decade ago, FDA was among the first to underscore that the science necessary to translate these discoveries into treatments—development of biomarkers, genomic data, modernized clinical trial designs, computer modeling, and advanced imaging technology—was not keeping pace. As a result, the process of drug development leading up to submission of a marketing application is often inefficient, costly, and slow.

What is needed to reduce the cost and length of drug development? Although no simple set of initiatives will quickly produce a flood of new treatments, much can be done to improve drug development, both in the short and long term. Today I want to talk about FDA's efforts to increase the speed and efficiency in several areas in the clinical trial phase of drug development. These include:

Accepting flexible clinical development designs; such flexible programs may use surrogate endpoints, or have fewer than the two traditional randomized, controlled trials of efficacy, or have other non-traditional elements.

Meeting frequently and working closely with industry sponsors throughout the development process to plan efficient clinical trial programs and agree on needed data, a process that has been shown to shorten drug development by up to several years.

Helping create clinical trial networks and "master protocols," where appropriate, to greatly reduce the cost of conducting clinical trials and reduce the time needed to carry them out.

- Using surrogate endpoints, both in accelerated approvals (approvals based on an unvalidated surrogate endpoint that is reasonably likely to predict clinical benefit) and traditional approvals (i.e., approvals not requiring confirmatory evidence of efficacy post- market). Surrogate endpoints have been the basis for 60 percent of rare-disease approvals.
- Listening carefully to patients and organizations that represent them to learn more about how they perceive benefits, risks, and unmet needs.
- When appropriate, encouraging the use of "adaptive" trial designs that allow design modifications as information about drug response accumulates, leading to more efficient studies.
- When appropriate, encouraging "enrichment" strategies to enroll patients more likely to respond to drugs under study, thereby reducing trial size and helping to direct drugs to patients who will benefit from them.
- Allowing the use of a wide range of study designs, including single-arm studies, when patient populations are extremely small, as in some orphan diseases, and the natural history of the disease is well-characterized and the drug's beneficial effects are large.
- Collaborating with scientists in industry and academia on biomarker development; and
- Identifying opportunities for streamlining regulatory processes.

I also want to point out some hurdles to efficient drug development, which require support for outside research and collaboration with other key stakeholders, including the National Institutes of Health (NIH), industry, and patient groups, to translate discoveries into treatments. These include basic research into a range of important diseases, such as Alzheimer's disease, whose causes are still poorly understood and for which drug development has proven particularly challenging.

FLEXIBLE TRIAL DESIGN

People with serious or life-threatening illnesses, particularly those who lack good alternatives, have told us repeatedly that they are willing to accept greater risks in order to gain access to new approved treatments.

FDA has long taken a flexible, rather than one-size-fits-all, approach to clinical trial design, urging that trials be designed as efficiently as possible to determine whether new drugs under investigation are safe and effective for their intended use, taking into account the severity and rarity of the disease and unmet need. A new study published in the *Journal of the American Medical Association* found that more than a third of 188 novel therapeutic drugs for 208 indications (uses) between 2005 and 2012 were approved on the basis of a single pivotal clinical trial, and in many cases, trials involved relatively small groups of patients for shorter durations.[1] All of this is possible, of course, when the drugs demonstrate strong beneficial effects.

Over 60 percent of drugs for rare diseases are approved on the basis of a single pivotal study, often because the cause of the disease is well understood and the pivotal study is supported by evidence of pertinent pharmacological effects, and because the natural history of untreated disease for many orphan conditions is well-characterized. All patients in such trials are given the new treatment, and the results are compared with the well-characterized natural history.[2] Thus, for example, last year, FDA approved Imbruvica (ibrutinib), a treatment for mantle cell lymphoma, based on an "open-label, single-arm trial," which means that every patient received the treatment and the trial was unblinded; i.e., both patients and researchers knew they were receiving the orphan drug under study. The results were compared to how well the 111 participating patients had responded to previous treatment for their disease. These designs are appropriate where there are objective responses (tumor shrinkage and recurrence, survival) where observational bias is limited, and where the natural history is clearly different from what treated patients experienced (tumors do not shrink spontaneously; survival is greatly increased).

In some cases, of course, small trials will not do the job. Some trials require large numbers of patients to demonstrate drug effects. This is often the case in studies of cardiovascular disease, where study endpoints, such as heart attack or stroke, while important, are not common.

Adaptive Trial Designs

FDA is also actively involved in developing adaptive trial designs, including designs with Bayesian adaptations based on interim assessments of biomarkers. Using this approach we try to find ways to adapt a clinical trial to the circumstances of the specific questions being asked in a way that is as efficient as possible but still gives us confidence in the results. The goal of these designs is to reduce trial duration and trial size. Importantly, these adaptations are performed with close attention to statistical rigor.

FDA is also conducting an internal research project to evaluate the amount and type of safety data required for new indications for cancer drugs. The goal is to identify ways to reduce the burden on sponsors, when submitting supplemental applications as well as regulatory review time, while ensuring patient safety. This research will be completed in November 2014.

Clinical Trial Enrichment

You also expressed interest in new tools to lower the cost of clinical trials. FDA issued guidance in December 2012 that explained how those developing drugs can use potentially powerful strategies to demonstrate a drug's effectiveness using clinical trial data.[3] Appropriate use of what we call clinical trial enrichment strategies could result in smaller studies, shortened drug development times, and lower development costs.

Working Closely with Drug Sponsors

As part of goals within the prescription drug user fee agreements included in the Food and Drug Administration Safety and Innovation Act (FDASIA), FDA works closely with sponsors of new drugs to design a development and review pathway for each drug that best reflects the disease and patients it is intended to treat, the drug itself, and other treatment options. Sponsors who avail themselves of the opportunity to meet with FDA early in development have substantially reduced the time from the start of human testing—when FDA first becomes involved—until marketing approval. For the 181 new drugs approved from 2008 - 2013 (for which a clinical development time could be calculated), the sponsors of the 67 applications who met with FDA before submitting their Investigational New Drug (IND) applications had a median development time of only 6.6 years, compared to 8.0 years for applications for which such a meeting did not occur (a mean reduction of 1.4 years). The median drug development time for applications for which a meeting with FDA was held at the end of the Phase 1 (EOP1) milestone was 1.1 years shorter than for applications for which an EOP1 meeting did not take place. For orphan drugs, drug development was a median of 2.1 years shorter.

In April 2014, we approved Zykadia (ceritinib), a new drug for patients with a certain type of late stage, non-small-cell lung cancer (NSCLC). It is one of four targeted therapies for lung cancer that have been approved since 2011—therapies that are the result of a new and forward-thinking approach to understanding the disease and its causes. FDA granted breakthrough designation to this drug, streamlining the development and review process with an "all hands on deck" approach. In fact, due to the enhanced understanding of how drugs like Zykadia work (by blocking anaplastic lymphoma kinase (ALK) and inhibiting the growth of lung cancer) and the frequent interactions between FDA and the drug's sponsor, it took less than four years—versus the roughly 10 years it used to take—from the initial study of the drug to FDA approval. This approval process exemplifies the strength of the collaborative process between FDA, industry, health advocacy organizations, and other stakeholders, while ensuring that FDA maintains its independent role in ensuring safety and efficiency of the product. And it illustrates the dedication and enthusiasm of FDA reviewers who carefully, but quickly, analyzed complex study results to allow for earlier approval and patient access to this new drug.

Surrogate Endpoints

The Accelerated Approval pathway allows for the use of surrogate endpoints, reasonably likely to predict a clinical benefit to get certain drugs for serious conditions more rapidly to patients. But many observers are not aware that FDA has also commonly used well-established surrogate endpoints for traditional approvals. Indeed, for the 94 new drugs approved by FDA between 2010 and 2012, 45 percent were approved on the basis of a surrogate endpoint. Once a surrogate is well established to predict clinical benefit, it can be used in traditional approvals and accelerated approval is no longer required. This saves time and the cost of the follow-up, confirmatory, clinical trial data collection required under accelerated approval.

For example, FDA regularly relies on a surrogate endpoint for approval of new therapies for diabetes, including several major new therapies in recent years, greatly expanding the physician's armamentarium for treating this disease. All were based on a well-established laboratory test (the HbA1C test, a measurement of hemoglobin with attached sugar in the blood that reflects the extent and persistence of elevated blood sugar) as a surrogate for clinical improvement, rather than requiring the sponsor to conduct decades-long studies to demonstrate an effect on long-term health. Moreover, it is critical that these endpoints are supported by sound science. As science evolves, we may discover that some of these endpoints are not accurate predictors and such discoveries are likewise critical.

Biomarkers and Targeted Drug Development

One of the most promising areas for advances in drug development is in predicting which patient populations will best respond to a new drug therapy, thereby enabling drug development to focus on the "subpopulation" most likely to benefit. This "targeted" approach is believed to be one of the keys to lowering drug development costs and expediting approval, at least for the population for which the drug can be quickly and effectively identified as a successful therapy. For example, within the last decade, the high-quality data submitted in applications and our collective understanding of the genetic and molecular underpinnings of lung cancer have enabled us to move from classifying the disease by what can be seen under a microscope to looking at the patient's molecular profile and classifying and treating the cancer by specific subtype. Scientists can now identify "driver oncogenes," which cause a normal cell to become cancerous and promote the growth of a patient's tumor. They can develop targeted therapies aimed at shutting down these aberrant genes and pathways—an example of an approach called personalized medicine. A targeted treatment is directed to the patients who will respond, while sparing others the potential for toxicity and delay in receiving other potentially effective treatments.

In the early 1990s, only 5 percent of FDA's new drug approvals were for targeted therapies. Twenty years later, that number had risen to a quarter of new approvals, and in 2013, 45 percent of FDA's approvals were for targeted therapies. Examples include several recently approved and important treatments for cancer, such as Mekinist, Tafinlar, Imbruvica, and Zykadia. The use of targeted therapies is expanding rapidly. Indeed, approximately 80 percent of new compounds FDA has designated as "breakthrough" therapies are targeted. Furthermore, accumulating evidence reveals that total development times for targeted therapies are up to two years less than for drugs aimed at broader treatment populations.

It is critical to understand, however, that our ability to use genomic data or to identify useful biomarkers depends on how well scientists understand the molecular and genetic causes and pathways of disease. The level of their understanding, in turn, depends on the strength of the foundational research into given diseases.

In some disease areas, we have made tremendous progress in our understanding of the causes of the disease and interventions that can treat or cure it. For example, decades of research on cancer and HIV/AIDS have given us critical insights into the pathways through which these (and related) diseases can be attacked, leading to discovery of biomarkers that predict disease progression as well as drug activity. Predicting likely progression allows selection of patients who will have many or earlier study endpoints, and thus use of fewer patients; predicting likelihood of response to treatment also allows for smaller studies and directs treatment to those who can benefit. FDA has been an active partner in developing and bringing therapies to market in these areas. This has resulted in important breakthroughs, rapid drug development, and a robust pipeline of new therapies.

However, the scientific community still lacks a complete understanding of the biology underlying disease such as Alzheimer's disease. As a result, many rational and well-intentioned approaches to develop disease biomarkers or surrogates for clinical endpoints have encountered unanticipated obstacles. While progress has been made on developing biomarkers for disease progression, these obstacles have made the development of biomarkers to assess drug activity difficult, and the treatment options for Alzheimer's disease remain extremely limited.

Scientific understanding of diseases varies widely and is likely to remain the most important limiting factor for developing targeted therapies and personalized medicine. When we do not understand the disease pathways, biomarkers appearing to be linked to disease progression often fail because they are not, in fact, in the causal pathway for the disease. The surprising Phase III failure of torcetrapib—Pfizer's would-be blockbuster to prevent heart attacks by raising HDL (the "good" cholesterol)—illustrates the risks of relying on an unvalidated, albeit seemingly reasonable, biomarker that turns out not to predict treatment outcomes.

MASTER PROTOCOLS AND CLINICAL TRIAL NETWORKS

One of the most serious limiting factors in drug development is the time and expenses required to design and conduct the Phase 3 clinical trials needed to demonstrate drug safety and effectiveness. As the President's Council of Advisors on Science and Technology (PCAST) observed in their 2012 report on drug innovation:

> Clinical trials constitute the largest single component of the R&D budget of the biopharmaceutical industry, at approximately $31.3 billion, representing nearly 40 percent of the R&D budget of major companies. Unfortunately, there is broad agreement that our current clinical trials system is inefficient. Currently, each clinical trial to test a new drug candidate is typically organized de novo, requiring substantial effort, cost, and time. . . . Navigating all of these requirements is challenging even for large pharmaceutical companies, and can be daunting for small biotechnology firms. Even in the best cases, the complexities add considerable time to trials—subtracting time from a successful drug's eventual time on the market without competition.[4]

Drug development need not necessarily be done in this way. There are often much better alternatives to reinventing the wheel every time a new clinical trial begins, including, where appropriate, the development of clinical trial networks and master protocols. The recently initiated Lung Cancer Master Protocol (Lung-MAP) is an excellent example of a new, less-costly paradigm for developing drugs, one that benefits both drug companies and patients. A master protocol creates a single clinical trial infrastructure that can test many drugs at the same time. Development of such a protocol requires close coordination with CDER reviewers, scientists in academia, NIH, and possibly other organizations, and the protocols themselves typically go through a peer review process. In the case of Lung-MAP, patients are assigned to one of five different drugs being simultaneously tested, based in part on their genetic profiles and their likelihood of responding to the study drug, and additional drugs can be added, while others are dropped, over time. The goal is to increase efficiencies through the use of a common biomarker screening platform, a common algorithm for assigning patients to multiple protocols ongoing concurrently, and the potential for sharing control patients across protocols for a given biomarker profile, all of which are possible because of the infrastructure established for the master protocol. FDA is highly supportive of master protocols.

PUBLIC-PRIVATE PARTNERSHIPS AND STAKEHOLDER ENGAGEMENT

Just like the September 2012 "Report on Propelling Innovation in Drug Discovery, Development, and Evaluation," from PCAST, FDA believes that bridging the gap between drug discovery and development can only be achieved through creative collaborations. Public-private partnerships enable stakeholders to leverage expertise and resources for the conduct of mutually beneficial research activities in the pre-competitive domain. And indeed, CDER is involved in at least 22 unique science-driven, public-private partnerships that promote development of research tools, platforms, clinical databases and predictive models to advance knowledge of disease and safety profiles of drugs. The recent approval of Zykadia, as mentioned earlier, for patients with a certain type of late-stage (metastatic) non-small-cell lung cancer, benefited from FDA's collaborative efforts with industry, health advocacy organizations, and others to identify the molecular underpinnings of cancer that would make it possible to classify and treat cancer by specific subtype.

FDA is also a partner in the Clinical Trials Transformation Initiative (CTTI)—a public-private partnership whose mission is to identify and promote practices that will increase the quality and efficiency of clinical trials. CTTI now comprises more than 60 organizations from across the clinical trial enterprise. Members include representatives of government agencies, industry representatives (pharmaceutical, biotech, device, and clinical research organizations), patient advocacy groups, professional societies, investigator groups, academic institutions, and other interested parties. CTTI is actively pursuing many new initiatives to reduce the time and cost of clinical trial programs, such as development of streamlined protocols and data collection recommendations for clinical trials of hospital-acquired bacterial pneumonia. Another example of a CTTI project with the potential to affect the clinical trial enterprise is its collaboration with FDA's Sentinel Initiative (Sentinel is FDA's active surveillance system that uses pre-existing electronic health care data from 18 data partners, capturing information on more than 150 million patient lives). A working group comprised of CTTI and Sentinel investigators is elucidating current barriers and identifying appropriate processes for the use of such electronic health care data to facilitate the conduct of clinical trials.

FDA also is partnering closely with many public-private initiatives, advocacy groups, and consortia. As one example, the Agency is a member of the recently announced NIH-led Accelerating Medicines Partnership (AMP), which is attempting to identify biological targets most likely to respond to new therapies and uncover biomarkers that may help predict clinical benefit in drug development in Alzhemier's disease, among others. FDA is working closely with the NIH's National Center for Advancing Translational Sciences (NCATS) to accelerate research on rare disease through NCATS' Innovative Therapeutics for Rare and Neglected Diseases program. We are also working with the Coalition Against Major Diseases (CAMD) to identify new tools and methods that can be applied to increase the efficiency of the development process of new treatments for Alzheimer's and Parkinson's diseases. The Agency's Drug Development Tool Qualification process also provides a mechanism to evaluate and qualify novel drug development tools (biomarkers, clinical outcome assessments, animal models under the Animal Rule) for an appropriate context of use. Recently, we deemed a "fit-for-purposed" drug development tool for Alzheimer's disease that CAMD has developed. These represent just a few of our many collaborations. See more at *http://blogs.fda.gov/fdavoice/index.php/page/5/#sthash.bWxzFv0M.dpuf.*

Lastly, FDA is engaged with TransCelerate Biopharma, Inc. (TCB), a non-profit organization established to facilitate pre-competitive collaboration among biopharma companies with the goal of accelerating the development of new medicines by identifying ways to make the clinical trial process more efficient. FDA is engaged in TCB's efforts to improve the conduct and efficiency of clinical trial sponsor oversight of clinical sites, clinical site qualification, and development of a common protocol template.

REGULATORY SCIENCE

The 21st century has seen rapid advances in biomedical research. New cutting-edge technologies have led to thousands of new drug candidates including: the sequencing of the human genome; combinatorial chemistry, a new method of chemical synthesis that makes it possible to prepare thousands of compounds in a single process; biosynthesis, which enables scientists to synthesize complex chemicals in living cells; and high throughput screening, which allows researchers to quickly conduct millions of genetic, chemical, or pharmacological tests. In addition, cutting-edge electronics and materials science have the power to transform medical devices, and research on nanotechnology-based materials will provide a better understanding of the safety of the use of nanomaterials in over-the-counter drugs. FDA's regulatory science research agenda is critical to help translate new technologies and basic science discoveries into safe and effective real-world diagnostics, treatments, and cures and to reduce the time, complexity, and cost of product development.

There can be no doubt that further modernizing and streamlining the science of how products are developed and evaluated is a complex challenge requiring new models and approaches that stress cross-sector and cross-disciplinary research. Advancing regulatory science has been one of FDA Commissioner Hamburg's key initiatives. New biomedical innovations may be enhanced by partnerships such as the Biomarkers Consortium, which promotes the development and qualification (or regulatory acceptance) of biomarkers (of which surrogate endpoints are a subset), using new and existing technologies.

CONSIDERATION OF ADDITIONAL APPROVAL PATHWAYS

PCAST also recommended the creation of a drug approval pathway under which sponsors could propose, early in the development process, to study a new drug for initial approval that would be reserved for use in a specific subgroup of patients that would allow a narrower development program than required for traditional approvals. While FDA has existing authority to approve products for subpopulations, in practice, drug development protocols generally evaluate drugs in a broader population, resulting in larger, lengthier trials. PCAST notes that a more clearly defined Special Medical Use or Limited Population pathway could encourage novel development programs for limited, well-defined subpopulations and complement FDA's existing efforts to get drugs to small, in-need populations faster. Such a pathway needs to consider the implications of market entry of a product for limited use. For example, an important consideration is how to encourage appropriate prescribing with the approved limited use for a specific population. Legislation focused on a pathway for drugs for serious or life-threatening bacterial and fungal infections in patients with unmet medical need—a particular area of unmet medical need highlighted in the PCAST report—has been introduced to address this issue, and we welcome the opportunity for continued discussions with stakeholders.

Having multiple approval pathways is important because they give drug sponsors options to help get therapies to patients needing them faster. Different pathways may also prove better for different products. In June 2013, less than one year after the enactment of the Food and Drug Administration Safety and Innovation Act (FDASIA), FDA issued draft guidance to bring more clarity to the accelerated approval program and other expedited programs for drugs and biologics that target serious conditions, so as to further encourage the use of these programs, *http://www.fda.gov/downloads/Drugs/GuidanceCompliance RegulatoryInformation/Guidances/UCM358301.pdf.* That guidance was finalized in May 2014. Although FDA has been able to speed the availability of drugs and biologics for serious conditions that provide a meaningful therapeutic benefit to patients over existing treatments under the accelerated approval program since 1992, FDASIA clarified that authority in legislation and emphasized FDA's ability to consider epidemiologic, pharmacologic, or other evidence developed using biomarkers or other scientific methods or tools in determining whether an endpoint can support accelerated approval.

Accelerated approval for drugs and biologics has been used primarily in settings in which the disease course is long and an extended period of time would be required to measure the intended clinical benefit of a drug or vaccine.

Further, the Agency oversees other programs that expedite the availability of new drugs for patients with serious conditions. For example, as part of FDASIA in 2012, Congress gave FDA new authority to designate drugs as breakthrough therapies. Breakthrough therapy designation is a program designed to expedite the development and review of drugs that are intended to treat a serious condition and which preliminary clinical evidence indicates may demonstrate substantial improvement over available therapy on one or more clinically significant endpoints. The breakthrough therapy program has already been well-utilized. As of June 13, 2014, CDER has received 164 requests for breakthrough therapy designation. CDER has granted breakthrough therapy designations for 48 of those requests, denied 83 such requests, and approved six breakthrough therapy drugs. CBER has had 31 breakthrough therapy designation requests, four of which it has granted and 26 of which it has denied.

FDA Efforts on Patient Engagement

In accordance with our commitments in the Prescription Drug User Fee Act of 2012 (PDUFA V), FDA has initiated the Patient-Focused Drug Development (PFDD) program. The objective of this five-year effort is to more systematically obtain the patient's perspective on a disease and its impact on patients' daily lives, the types of treatment benefit that matter most to patients, and the adequacy of available therapies for the disease. As part of this commitment, FDA is holding at least 20 public meetings over the course of PDUFA V; each of which will focus on a specific disease area. We have already held patient meetings on several major diseases.

After conducting a public process to nominate disease areas for Fiscal Years 2013-2015, FDA held the first PFDD meeting on April 25, 2013. This meeting focused on chronic fatigue syndrome (CFS) and myalgic encephalomyelitis (ME), sometimes called CFS-ME, a debilitating disease for which there are currently no FDA-approved treatments.

Here, we heard directly from patients, patient advocates, and caretakers about the symptoms that matter most to them, the impact the disease has on patients' daily lives, and the patient experience with currently available treatments. FDA staff, including members of FDA's Division of Pulmonary, Allergy, and Rheumatology Products, listened carefully to the personal accounts of this devastating condition.

After the meeting, we released a report titled *The Voice of the Patient: Chronic Fatigue Syndrome and Myalgic Encephalomyeliti*, a detailed summary of the meeting. In this report we documented, in the patients' own words, what disease impacts and treatment approaches mattered most to them. This summary included patient testimony at the meeting, perspectives shared in 230 docket comments, as well as unique views provided those joining the meeting via webcast. Moreover, on March 11, 2014, FDA also released draft guidance (found at *http://www.fda.gov/downloads/Drugs/GuidanceCompliance Regu latoryInformation/Guidances/U CM388568.pdf)* for industry entitled "*Chronic Fatigue Syndrome/Myalgic Encephalomyelitis:*

Developing Drug Products for Treatment." The purpose of the guidance is to assist sponsors in developing drug products for the treatment of CFS-ME.

The PFDD reports, such as the one developed after the CFS-ME meeting, will serve an important function in communicating to both FDA review staff and the regulated industry what improvements patients would most like to see in their daily lives. These reports will strengthen the structured framework for benefit-risk assessment in the new drug process, which FDASIA (Sec. 905) requires and which is currently in development, that will be used to help communicate patients' values to the FDA review team during product review. FDA believes that the long-term impact of the PFDD program will be a better, more informed understanding of how the entire drug development community might find ways to develop new treatments for diseases.

Soon after the CFS and ME meeting, in June 2013, we conducted similar meetings on HIV and lung cancer, and the summary reports are now available on our website. The reports for our recent meetings on narcolepsy and sickle cell disease will be posted soon. We have also held meetings on fibromyalgia, pulmonary arterial hypertension, and metabolism.

By the end of FY 2015, we plan to have conducted at least 16 PFDD meetings to hear from patients suffering from and living with a wide range of conditions. These are currently identified on our webpage: *http://www.fda.gov/ForIndustry/UserFees/PrescriptionDrugUserFee/ucm347317.htm.* For the remaining two years in PDUFA V, we will conduct another public process to identify the diseases that will be addressed during that time.

We are gratified by the enthusiastic response within the patient community to PFDD, and we look forward to continued input from these meetings—and to the long-term benefit they can offer for drug development in important therapeutic areas.

In addition to these efforts, CDER established the Professional Affairs and Stakeholder Engagement program that will serve as a focal point and enhance two-way communications and collaboration with health professional organizations and patient advocacy and consumer groups about drug products.

Conclusion

FDA welcomes the opportunity to constructively engage and work with Congress and stakeholders in an effort to improve review efficiency and effectiveness while maintaining the high safety and efficacy standards for which FDA approval has become the global "gold standard."

Thank you for the opportunity to testify today. I am happy to answer any questions.

End Notes

[1] Downing NS, Aminawung JA, Shah ND, Krumholz HM, Ross JS. Clinical Trial Evidence Supporting FDA Approval of Novel Therapeutic Agents, 2005-2012. JAMA, 2014; 311(4): 368-377.

[2] Sasinowski FJ. Quantum of effectiveness evidence in FDA's approval of orphan drugs. Drug Information J. 2012; 46:238-63.

[3] Guidance for Industry: Enrichment Strategies for Clinical Trials to Support Approval of Human Drugs and Biological Products. December 2012 http://www.fda.gov/downloads/Drugs/GuidanceComplianceRegulatoryInformation/Guidances/UCM332181.pdf.

[4] "Report to the President on Propelling Innovation in Drug Discovery, Development and Evaluation," President's Council of 13 Advisors on Science and Technology, The White House, Washington, D.C., September, 2012, p. 20.

In: FDA's Expedited Drug Programs
Editor: Gary Lawrence
ISBN: 978-1-63485-772-7

Chapter 3

GUIDANCE FOR INDUSTRY: EXPEDITED PROGRAMS FOR SERIOUS CONDITIONS – DRUGS AND BIOLOGICS*

Food and Drug Administration

This guidance represents the Food and Drug Administration's (FDA's) current thinking on this topic. It does not create or confer any rights for or on any person and does not operate to bind FDA or the public. You can use an alternative approach if the approach satisfies the requirements of the applicable statutes and regulations. If you want to discuss an alternative approach, contact the FDA staff responsible for implementing this guidance. If you cannot identify the appropriate FDA staff, call the appropriate number listed at the end of this guidance.

I. INTRODUCTION

The following four FDA programs are intended to facilitate and expedite development and review of new drugs[2] to address unmet medical need in the treatment of a serious or lifethreatening[3] condition: fast track designation, breakthrough therapy designation, accelerated approval, and priority review designation (see section IV for an overview of the programs). The purpose of

* This is an edited, reformatted and augmented version of document issued by the U.S. Department of Health and Human Services, May 2014.

this guidance for industry is to provide a single resource for information on FDA's policies and procedures for these four programs as well as threshold criteria generally applicable to concluding that a drug is a candidate for these expedited development and review programs.

FDA's guidance documents, including this guidance, do not establish legally enforceable responsibilities. Instead, guidances describe the Agency's current thinking on a topic and should be viewed only as recommendations, unless specific regulatory or statutory requirements are cited. The use of the word *should* in Agency guidances means that something is suggested or recommended, but not required.

II. BACKGROUND

The programs described in this guidance are intended to help ensure that therapies for serious conditions are approved and available to patients as soon as it can be concluded that the therapies' benefits justify their risks. The Agency first formally articulated its thinking on expediting the availability of promising new therapies in regulations codified at part 312, subpart E (21 CFR part 312).[4] The subpart E regulations are intended to speed the availability of new therapies to patients with serious conditions, especially when there are no satisfactory alternative therapies, while preserving appropriate standards for safety and effectiveness. The regulations call for earlier attention to drugs that have promise in treating such conditions, including early consultation with FDA for sponsors of such products and efficient trial design, potentially relying on well-controlled phase 2 studies for evidence of effectiveness. The subpart E regulations specifically recognize that patients and physicians are generally willing to accept greater risks and side effects from treatment of life-threatening and severely debilitating diseases than they would for other diseases. The four principal programs that support these principles are fast track designation, breakthrough therapy designation, accelerated approval, and priority review designation (referred to in this guidance as the Agency's *expedited programs*).

FDA has a history of applying the philosophy underlying subpart E to drugs for rare diseases through use of the Agency's expedited programs. FDA recognizes that certain aspects of drug development that are feasible for common diseases may not be feasible for rare diseases and that development challenges are often greater with increasing rarity of the disease. FDA will continue to apply flexibility in these situations to address particular challenges posed by each disease.

III. Concepts for Expedited Programs

The programs that are the subject of this guidance, fast track designation, breakthrough therapy designation, accelerated approval, and priority review, are summarized in section IV and described individually in detail in sections V, VI, VII, and VIII. All four expedited programs represent efforts to address an unmet medical need in the treatment of a serious condition, which is discussed in the following paragraphs.

A. Serious Condition

1. Whether a Condition Is Serious

FDA intends to interpret the term *serious* as it has done in the past for the purposes of accelerated approval[5] and expanded access to investigational drugs for treatment use.[6] A serious disease or condition is defined in the expanded access regulations as follows:

> . . . a disease or condition associated with morbidity that has substantial impact on day-to-day functioning. Short-lived and self-limiting morbidity will usually not be sufficient, but the morbidity need not be irreversible if it is persistent or recurrent. Whether a disease or condition is serious is a matter of clinical judgment, based on its impact on such factors as survival, day-to-day functioning, or the likelihood that the disease, if left untreated, will progress from a less severe condition to a more serious one.[7]
>
> Note: For the purposes of this guidance, the terms *condition, disease*, and *illness* are used interchangeably. All conditions meeting the definition of life-threatening as set forth at § 312.81(a) would also be serious conditions.

2. Whether the Drug Is Intended to Treat a Serious Condition

As referenced in section IV, the statutory and regulatory eligibility criteria for expedited programs require that a drug be intended to treat a serious condition. To satisfy this criterion, a drug must be intended to have an effect on a serious condition or a serious aspect of a condition, such as a direct effect on a serious manifestation or symptom of a condition or other intended effects, including the following:

- A diagnostic product intended to improve diagnosis or detection of a serious condition in a way that would lead to improved outcomes.
- A product intended to mitigate or prevent a serious treatment-related side effect (e.g., serious infections in patients receiving immunosuppressive therapy).
- A product intended to avoid or diminish a serious adverse event associated with available therapy for a serious condition (e.g., product that is less cardiotoxic than available cancer therapy)[8].
- A product intended to prevent a serious condition or reduce the likelihood that the condition will progress to a more serious condition or a more advanced stage of disease.

B. Available Therapy

For purposes of this guidance, FDA generally considers *available therapy* (and the terms *existing treatment* and *existing therapy*) as a therapy that:

- Is approved or licensed in the United States for the same indication being considered for the new drug[9] and
- Is relevant to current U.S. standard of care (SOC) for the indication

FDA's available therapy determination generally focuses on treatment options that reflect the current SOC for the specific indication (including the disease stage) for which a product is being developed. In evaluating the current SOC, FDA considers recommendations by authoritative scientific bodies (e.g., National Comprehensive Cancer Network, American Academy of Neurology) based on clinical evidence and other reliable information that reflects current clinical practice. When a drug development program targets a subset of a broader disease population (e.g., a subset identified by a genetic mutation), the SOC for the broader population, if there is one, generally is considered available therapy for the subset, unless there is evidence that the SOC is less effective in the subset.

Over the course of new drug development, it is foreseeable that the SOC for a given condition may evolve (e.g., because of approval of a new therapy or new information about available therapies). FDA will determine what constitutes available therapy at the time of the relevant regulatory decision for each expedited program a sponsor intends to use (e.g., generally early in development for fast track and breakthrough therapy designations, at time of biologics license application (BLA) or new drug application (NDA) submissions for priority review designation, during BLA or NDA review for accelerated approval). FDA encourages sponsors to discuss available therapy considerations with the Agency during interactions with FDA.

As appropriate, FDA may consult with special Government employees or other experts when making an available therapy determination.

When determining whether a drug granted accelerated approval or approved with a risk evaluation and mitigation strategy (REMS) that includes elements to assure safe use (ETASU) under section 505-1 of the Federal Food, Drug, and Cosmetic Act (FD&C Act) (21 U.S.C. 355- 1), is considered available therapy, the following principles will be applied:

- A drug would not be considered available therapy if the drug is granted accelerated approval based on a surrogate endpoint or an intermediate clinical endpoint and clinical benefit has not been verified by postapproval studies. (See section III.C.3.)
- A drug would be considered available therapy if the drug is granted accelerated approval because of restricted distribution and the study population for the new drug under development is eligible to receive the approved drug under the restricted distribution program. Similarly, a drug would be considered available therapy if the study population for the new drug under development is eligible to receive the approved drug under the ETASU REMS.

C. Unmet Medical Need

An unmet medical need is a condition whose treatment or diagnosis is not addressed adequately by available therapy. An unmet medical need includes an immediate need for a defined population (i.e., to treat a serious condition with no or limited treatment) or a longer-term need for society (e.g., to address the development of resistance to antibacterial drugs).

1. Where There Is No Available Therapy

If there is no available therapy for a serious condition, there is clearly an unmet medical need.

2. Where There Is Available Therapy

When available therapy exists for a condition, a new treatment generally would be considered to address an unmet medical need if the treatment:

- Has an effect on a serious outcome of the condition that is not known to be influenced by available therapy (e.g., progressive disability or disease progression when the available therapy has shown an effect on symptoms, but has not shown an effect on progressive disability or disease progression)
- Has an improved effect on a serious outcome(s) of the condition compared with available therapy (e.g., superiority of the new drug to available therapy when either used alone or in combination with available therapy (i.e., as demonstrated in an add-on study))
- Has an effect on a serious outcome of the condition in patients who are unable to tolerate or failed to respond to available therapy
- Can be used effectively with other critical agents that cannot be combined with available therapy
- Provides efficacy comparable to those of available therapy, while (1) avoiding serious toxicity that occurs with available therapy, (2) avoiding less serious toxicity that is common and causes discontinuation of treatment of a serious condition, or (3) reducing the potential for harmful drug interactions
- Provides safety and efficacy comparable to those of available therapy but has a documented benefit, such as improved compliance, that is expected to lead to an improvement in serious outcomes
- Addresses an emerging or anticipated public health need, such as a drug shortage

In some disease settings, a drug that is not shown to provide a direct efficacy or safety advantage over available therapy may nonetheless provide an advantage that would be of sufficient public health benefit to qualify as meeting an unmet medical need. For example, in a condition for which there are approved therapies that have a modest response rate or significant heterogeneity in response, a drug with a novel mechanism of action (but comparable safety and effectiveness) could have the potential to provide an advantage over available therapy in some patients. In such a case, the novel mechanism of action should have a well-understood relationship to the disease pathophysiology. In addition, there should be a reasonable basis for concluding that a significant number of patients may respond differently to the new drug compared with available therapy. Thus, mechanistic diversity, even without a documented efficacy or safety advantage, could be advantageous in disease settings in which drugs become less effective or ineffective over time.

For example, infectious disease drugs or targeted cancer therapies with novel mechanisms of action, although appearing to have efficacy similar to available therapy across the disease population, could benefit patients who no longer respond to available therapy. Accordingly, FDA intends to consider a range of potential advantages over available therapy beyond those shown in head-to-head comparisons.

3. Where the Only Available Therapy Was Approved under the Accelerated Approval Program Based on a Surrogate Endpoint or an Intermediate Clinical Endpoint and Clinical Benefit Has Not Yet Been Verified

As discussed in sections VII and III.B., FDA recognizes, as a general matter, that it is preferable to have more than one treatment approved under the accelerated approval provisions because of the possibility that clinical benefit may not be verified in postapproval confirmatory trials. FDA will therefore consider products as addressing an unmet medical need if the only approved treatments were granted accelerated approval based on a surrogate endpoint or an intermediate clinical endpoint and clinical benefit has not been verified by postapproval studies.

IV. Overview of Expedited Programs

The table provides an overview of the four expedited programs. Additional details on the specific programs are found in the sections that follow. Note that a drug development program may qualify for more than one expedited program.

Comparison of FDA's Expedited Programs for Serious Conditions

	Fast Track	**Breakthrough Therapy**	**Accelerated Approval**	**Priority Review**
Nature of program	Designation	Designation	Approval Pathway	Designation
Reference	• Section 506(b) of the FD&C Act, as added by section 112 of the Food and Drug Administration Modernization Act of 1997 (FDAMA) and amended by section 901 of the Food and Drug Administration Safety and Innovation Act of 2012 (FDASIA)	• Section 506(a) of the FD&C Act, as added by section 902 of FDASIA	• 21 CFR part 314, subpart H • 21 CFR part 601, subpart E • Section 506(c) of the FD&C Act, as amended by section 901 of FDASIA	• Prescription Drug User Fee Act of 1992
Qualifying criteria	• A drug that is intended to treat a serious condition **AND** nonclinical or clinical data demonstrate the potential to address unmet medical need **OR** • A drug that has been designated as a qualified infectious disease product[a]	• A drug that is intended to treat a serious condition **AND** preliminary clinical evidence indicates that the drug may demonstrate substantial improvement on a clinically significant endpoint(s) over available therapies	• A drug that treats a serious condition **AND** generally provides a meaningful advantage over available therapies **AND** demonstrates an effect on a surrogate endpoint that is reasonably likely to predict clinical benefit or on a clinical endpoint that can be measured earlier than irreversible morbidity or mortality (IMM) that is	• An application (original or efficacy supplement) for a drug that treats a serious condition **AND,** if approved, would provide a significant improvement in safety or effectiveness **OR** • Any supplement that proposes a labeling change pursuant to a report on a pediatric study under 505A[b] **OR**

	Fast Track	Breakthrough Therapy	Accelerated Approval	Priority Review
Nature of program	Designation	Designation	Approval Pathway	Designation
			reasonably likely to predict an effect on IMM or other clinical benefit (i.e., an intermediate clinical endpoint)	• An application for a drug that has been designated as a qualified infectious disease product[c] **OR** • Any application or supplement for a drug submitted with a priority review voucher[d]
When to submit request	• With IND or after • Ideally, no later than the pre-BLA or pre-NDA meeting	• With IND or after • Ideally, no later than the end-of-phase 2 meeting	• The sponsor should ordinarily discuss the possibility of accelerated approval with the review division during development, supporting, for example, the use of the planned endpoint as a basis for approval and discussing the confirmatory trials, which should usually be already underway at the time of approval	• With original BLA, NDA, or efficacy supplement
Timelines for FDA response	• Within 60 calendar days of receipt of the request	• Within 60 calendar days of receipt of the request	• Not specified	• Within 60 calendar days of receipt of original BLA, NDA, or efficacy supplement
Features	• Actions to expedite development and review • Rolling review	• Intensive guidance on efficient drug development • Organizational commitment	• Approval based on an effect on a surrogate endpoint or an intermediate clinical endpoint that is reasonably likely to predict a drug's clinical benefit	• Shorter clock for review of marketing application (6 months compared with the 10-month standard review)[e]

(Continued)

	Fast Track	Breakthrough Therapy	Accelerated Approval	Priority Review
Nature of program	Designation	Designation	Approval Pathway	Designation
		• Rolling review • Other actions to expedite review		
Additional considerations	• Designation may be rescinded if it no longer meets the qualifying criteria for fast track[f]	• Designation may be rescinded if it no longer meets the qualifying criteria for breakthrough therapy[g]	• Promotional materials • Confirmatory trials to verify and describe the anticipated effect on IMM or other clinical benefit • Subject to expedited withdrawal	• Designation will be assigned at the time of original BLA, NDA, or efficacy supplement filing

[a] Title VIII of FDASIA, *Generating Antibiotic Incentives Now (GAIN),* provides incentives for the development of antibacterial and antifungal drugs for human use intended to treat serious and life threatening infections. Under GAIN, a drug may be designated as a *qualified infectious disease product (QIDP)* if it meets the criteria outlined in the statute. A drug that receives QIDP designation is eligible under the statute for fast track designation and priority review. However, QIDP designation is beyond the scope of this guidance.

[b] Any supplement to an application under section 505 of the FD&C Act that proposes a labeling change pursuant to a report on a pediatric study under this section shall be considered a priority review supplement per section 505A of the FD&C Act as amended by section 5(b) of the Best Pharmaceuticals for Children Act.

[c] See footnote a above.

[d] Any application or supplement that is submitted with a priority review voucher will be assigned a priority review. Priority review vouchers will be granted to applicants of applications for drugs for the treatment or prevention of certain tropical diseases, as defined in section 524(a)(3) and (a)(4) of the FD&C Act and for treatment of rare pediatric diseases as defined in section 529(a)(3) of the FD&C Act.

[e] As part of its commitments in PDUFA V, FDA has established a review model, *the Program.* The Program applies to all new molecular entity NDAs and original BLAs, including applications that are resubmitted following a Refuse-to-File action, received from October 1, 2012, through September 30, 2017. For applications filed by FDA under the Program, the PDUFA review clock will begin at the conclusion of the 60 calendar day filing review period that begins on the date of FDA receipt of the original submission.

[f] A sponsor may also withdraw fast track designation if the designation is no longer supported by emerging data or the drug development program is no longer being pursued (see section A.5. of Appendix 1).

[g] A sponsor may also withdraw breakthrough therapy designation if the designation is no longer supported by emerging data or the drug development program is no longer being pursued (see section B.5. of Appendix 1).

V. Fast Track Designation

Section 506(b) of the FD&C Act provides for the designation of a drug as a fast track product ". . . if it is intended, whether alone or in combination with one or more other drugs, for the treatment of a serious or life-threatening disease or condition, and it demonstrates the potential to address unmet medical needs for such a disease or condition." This provision is intended to facilitate development and expedite review of drugs to treat serious and life-threatening conditions so that an approved product can reach the market expeditiously. This section describes the qualifying criteria and the features of fast track designation. Appendix 1 describes the process for fast track designation.

A. Qualifying Criteria for Fast Track Designation

Fast track designation applies to the drug (either alone or in combination with other drugs) and the specific use for which it is being studied. The term *drug* refers to the combination of two or more drugs if the combination is the subject of the fast track designation or request. Where appropriate, FDA may grant designation to the development of a new use of an approved drug.

1. Serious Condition

See section III.A.

2. Demonstrating the Potential to Address Unmet Medical Need

The type of information needed to demonstrate the potential of a drug to address an unmet medical need will depend on the stage of drug development at which fast track designation is requested. Early in development, evidence of activity in a nonclinical model, a mechanistic rationale, or pharmacologic data could be used to demonstrate such potential. Later in development, available clinical data should demonstrate the potential to address an unmet medical need. See section III.C.

B. Features of Fast Track Designation

1. Actions to Expedite Development and Review

There are opportunities for frequent interactions with the review team for a fast track product. These include meetings with FDA, including pre-IND meetings, end-of-phase 1 meetings, and end-of-phase 2 meetings to discuss study design, extent of safety data required to support approval, dose-response concerns, and use of biomarkers. Other meetings may be scheduled as appropriate (e.g., to discuss accelerated approval, the structure and content of an NDA, and other critical issues).

In addition, such a product could be eligible for priority review if supported by clinical data at the time of BLA, NDA, or efficacy supplement submission (see section VIII).

2. Submission of Portions of an Application (Rolling Review)

If FDA determines, after preliminary evaluation of clinical data submitted by a sponsor, that a fast track product may be effective, the Agency may consider reviewing portions of a marketing application before the sponsor submits the complete application (see Appendix 2).[10]

VI. BREAKTHROUGH THERAPY DESIGNATION

Section 506(a) of the FD&C Act provides for designation of a drug as a breakthrough therapy ". . . if the drug is intended, alone or in combination with 1 or more other drugs, to treat a serious or life-threatening disease or condition and preliminary clinical evidence indicates that the drug may demonstrate substantial improvement over existing therapies on 1 or more clinically significant endpoints, such as substantial treatment effects observed early in clinical development." It is important to recognize that the standard for breakthrough therapy designation is not the same as the standard for drug approval. The clinical evidence needed to support breakthrough designation is preliminary. In contrast, as is the case for all drugs, FDA will review the full data submitted to support approval of drugs designated as breakthrough therapies to determine whether the drugs are safe and effective for their intended use before they are approved for marketing. This section describes the qualifying criteria and the features of breakthrough therapy designation. Appendix 1 describes the process for breakthrough therapy designation.

Not all products designated as breakthrough therapies ultimately will be shown to have the substantial improvement over available therapies suggested by the preliminary clinical evidence at the time of designation. If the designation is no longer supported by subsequent data, FDA may rescind the designation.[11] Because FDA commits significant resources to work particularly closely with sponsors of breakthrough therapy products, the Agency needs to focus its resources on breakthrough therapy drug development programs that continue to meet the program's qualifying criteria (see section B.5. in Appendix 1).

A. Qualifying Criteria for Breakthrough Therapy Designation

Breakthrough therapy designation applies to the drug (either alone or in combination with other drugs) and the specific use for which it is being studied. The term *drug* refers to the combination of two or more drugs if the combination is the subject of the breakthrough therapy designation or request. Where appropriate, FDA may grant designation to the development of a new use of an approved drug.

1. Serious Condition

See section III.A.

2. Existing (or Available) Therapies

See section III.B.

3. Preliminary Clinical Evidence

Unlike the information that could support fast track designation, which could include theoretical rationale, mechanistic rationale (based on nonclinical data), or evidence of nonclinical activity, breakthrough therapy designation requires preliminary clinical evidence of a treatment effect that may represent substantial improvement over available therapies for the treatment of a serious condition. For purposes of breakthrough therapy designation, *preliminary clinical evidence* means evidence that is sufficient to indicate that the drug may demonstrate substantial improvement in effectiveness or safety over available therapies, but in most cases is not sufficient to establish safety and effectiveness for purposes of approval. FDA expects that such evidence generally would be derived from phase 1 or 2 trials. Nonclinical information could support the clinical evidence of drug activity. In all cases, preliminary clinical evidence demonstrating that the drug may represent a substantial improvement over available therapy should involve a sufficient number of patients to be considered credible. However, FDA recognizes that the data cannot be expected to be definitive at the time of designation.

Ideally, preliminary clinical evidence indicating a substantial improvement over available therapies would be derived from a study that compares the investigational drug to an available therapy (or placebo, if there is no available therapy) in clinical testing or from a study that compares the new treatment plus SOC to the SOC alone. FDA encourages sponsors to obtain some preliminary comparative data of this type early in development. Other types of clinical data that also could be persuasive include single-arm studies comparing the new treatment with well-documented historical experience. Generally, FDA expects that such historically controlled data would be persuasive only if there is a large difference between the new treatment and historical experience. For example, where lung function decline is a major manifestation of a disease, single-arm study data showing that a new drug significantly increases lung function could be persuasive if there is no available therapy that increases lung function. Data demonstrating that a cancer drug substantially increases overall response rate compared with historical controls (e.g., historical response rate with available therapy), with consideration of duration of the response, also could be persuasive. Sponsors contemplating the use of historical controls should consult FDA's ICH guidance for industry *E10 Choice of Control Group and Related Issues in Clinical Trials* for more-detailed discussions.[12]

4. May Demonstrate Substantial Improvement on Clinically Significant Endpoint(s)

To support a breakthrough therapy designation, the preliminary clinical evidence must show that the drug may demonstrate substantial improvement over available therapy on one or more clinically significant endpoints.

Substantial Improvement: The determination of whether the improvement over available therapy is substantial is a matter of judgment and depends on both the magnitude of the drug's effect on a clinically significant endpoint (which could include duration of the effect) and the importance of the observed effect to the treatment of the serious condition or serious aspect of the condition. In general, the preliminary clinical evidence should show a clear advantage over available therapy.

Approaches to demonstrating substantial improvement include the following:

- Direct comparison of the new drug to available therapy shows a much greater or more important response (e.g., complete responses where the control treatment generally results only in partial responses). Such a trial could be conducted in treatment-naïve patients or in those whose disease failed to respond to available therapies, either as a comparison with the failed therapy (if ethically acceptable) or as a no-treatment controlled study.
- If there is no available therapy, the new drug shows a substantial and clinically meaningful effect on an important outcome when compared with a placebo or a well-documented historical control.
- The new drug added to available therapy results in a much greater or more important response compared to available therapy in a controlled study or to a well-documented historical control. This trial also could be conducted in treatment-naïve patients or in those whose disease failed to respond to available therapies.
- The new drug has a substantial and clinically meaningful effect on the underlying cause of the disease, in contrast to available therapies that treat only symptoms of the disease, and preliminary clinical evidence indicates that the drug is likely to have a disease-modifying effect in the long term (e.g., a sustained clinical benefit compared with a temporary clinical benefit provided by available therapies).
- The new drug reverses or inhibits disease progression, in contrast to available therapies that only provide symptomatic improvement.
- The new drug has an important safety advantage that relates to serious adverse reactions (e.g., those that may result in treatment interruption) compared with available therapies and has similar efficacy.

Clinically Significant Endpoint: For purposes of breakthrough therapy designation, FDA considers clinically significant endpoint generally to refer to an endpoint that measures an effect on irreversible morbidity or mortality (IMM) or on symptoms that represent serious consequences of the disease. It can also refer to findings that suggest an effect on IMM or serious symptoms, including:

- An effect on an established surrogate endpoint that typically would be used to support traditional approval

- An effect on a surrogate endpoint or intermediate clinical endpoint (see section VII.B.2.) considered reasonably likely to predict a clinical benefit (i.e., the accelerated approval standard)
- A significantly improved safety profile compared with available therapy (e.g., less dose-limiting toxicity for an oncology agent), with evidence of similar efficacy

In a breakthrough therapy designation request, a sponsor should provide justification for why the endpoint or other findings should be considered clinically significant.

In rare cases, a pharmacodynamic (PD) biomarker may be considered a clinically significant endpoint if it strongly suggests the potential for a clinically meaningful effect on the underlying disease. In such cases, a sponsor should provide evidence supporting the use of the PD biomarker. Such evidence should include, for example, (1) the extent of understanding of the disease pathophysiology, (2) whether the biomarker is on a causal pathway of the disease process, and (3) the time course of the drug's effect on the biomarker (e.g., the biomarker can be measured earlier than a surrogate endpoint used for accelerated approval). In addition, strong evidence of the drug's effect on the PD biomarker generally is expected. FDA is more likely to rely on a PD biomarker for breakthrough therapy designation in a disease setting in which there is no available therapy, if the evidence supports such use.

B. Features of Breakthrough Therapy Designation

1. Intensive Guidance on an Efficient Drug Development Program, Beginning as Early as Phase 1

As discussed previously, breakthrough therapy designation will usually mean that the effect of the drug will be large compared with available therapies. In such cases, the development program for the breakthrough therapy could be considerably shorter than for other drugs intended to treat the disease being studied. However, FDA notes that a compressed drug development program still must generate adequate data to demonstrate that the drug is safe and effective to meet the statutory standard for approval.[13] Omitting components of the drug development program that are necessary for such a determination can significantly delay, or even preclude, marketing approval.

Sponsors can design efficient clinical trials in a number of ways. FDA will seek to ensure that a sponsor of a product designated as a breakthrough therapy receives timely advice and interactive communications to help the sponsor design and conduct a drug development program as efficiently as possible.[14] During these interactions, the Agency may suggest, or a sponsor may propose, alternative clinical trial designs (e.g., adaptive designs, an enrichment strategy, crossover or N-of-1 design, use of historical controls) or use of an interim analysis by a data monitoring committee.[15] These trial designs may result in smaller trials or more efficient trials that require less time to complete and may help minimize the number of patients exposed to a potentially less efficacious treatment (i.e., the control group treated with available therapy). Such approaches may be especially useful in studies in rare diseases. For example, single-arm trials may be an important option in rare diseases with well-understood pathophysiology and a well-defined disease course.

FDA anticipates that the review team and the sponsor will meet and interact throughout drug development to address these and other important issues at different phases of development. In addition, a sponsor should be prepared for a more rapid pace for other aspects of the drug development (e.g., manufacturing (see section IX.A.), development of a necessary companion diagnostic (see section IX.D.)).

2. Organizational Commitment Involving Senior Managers

FDA intends to expedite the development and review of a breakthrough therapy by intensively involving senior managers and experienced review and regulatory health project management staff in a proactive, collaborative, cross-disciplinary review. Where appropriate, FDA also intends to assign a cross-disciplinary project lead for the review team to facilitate an efficient review of the drug development program. The cross-disciplinary project lead will serve as a scientific liaison between members of the review team (e.g., medical; clinical pharmacology; pharmacology-toxicology; chemistry, manufacturing, and controls (CMC); compliance; biostatistics), facilitating coordinated internal interactions and communications with a sponsor through the review division's regulatory health project manager.

3. Submission of Portions of an Application (Rolling Review)

FDA has determined that it is appropriate for a drug designated as a breakthrough therapy to be able to obtain rolling review. Therefore, if FDA determines, after preliminary evaluation of clinical data submitted by the sponsor, that a breakthrough therapy product may be effective, the Agency may consider reviewing portions of a marketing application before the sponsor submits the complete application (see Appendix 2).

4. Other Actions to Expedite Review

In addition, such a product could be eligible for priority review if supported by clinical data at the time of BLA, NDA, or efficacy supplement submission.

VII. ACCELERATED APPROVAL

The accelerated approval provisions of FDASIA in section 506(c) of the FD&C Act provide that FDA may grant accelerated approval to:

> . . . a product for a serious or life-threatening disease or condition . . . upon a determination that the product has an effect on a surrogate endpoint that is reasonably likely to predict clinical benefit, or on a clinical endpoint that can be measured earlier than irreversible morbidity or mortality, that is reasonably likely to predict an effect on irreversible morbidity or mortality or other clinical benefit, taking into account the severity, rarity, or prevalence of the condition and the availability or lack of alternative treatments.

For drugs granted accelerated approval, postmarketing confirmatory trials have been required to verify and describe the anticipated effect on IMM or other clinical benefit (see sections VII.D.2. and VII.D.3.).[16]

This section describes the qualifying criteria, relevant terms, and the conditions of accelerated approval. The provisions of FDASIA facilitate somewhat broader use of accelerated approval to expedite patients' access to important treatments for serious conditions. FDA believes the new provisions provide additional flexibility concerning the implications of available therapy on eligibility for accelerated approval (see section VII.A.2.). They also provide clarification concerning the use of clinical endpoints (herein referred to as intermediate clinical endpoints) as a basis for accelerated approval (see section VII.B.2.). In addition, the new provisions make clear that FDA has the authority to consider pharmacologic or other evidence developed using biomarkers or other scientific methods or tools, in conjunction with other data, in determining whether an endpoint is reasonably likely to predict clinical benefit (see section VII.C.).[17] By indicating that FDA should take into account, ". . . the severity, rarity, or prevalence of the condition . . ." in considering whether to grant accelerated approval, FDASIA reinforces the Agency's longstanding commitment to regulatory flexibility regarding the evidence required to support product approval for the treatment of serious or life-threatening diseases with limited therapeutic options.

The accelerated approval pathway has been used primarily in settings in which the disease course is long and an extended period of time would be required to measure the intended clinical benefit of a drug. For example, accelerated approval has been used extensively in the approval of drugs to treat a variety of cancers and human immunodeficiency virus (HIV) disease where an effect on tumor growth or viral load can be assessed rapidly, but demonstrating an effect on survival or morbidity generally requires lengthy and sometimes large trials because of the duration of the typical disease course. Accelerated approval is also potentially useful in acute disease settings where the intended clinical benefit can be demonstrated only in a very large study because the clinical event that would need to be evaluated to demonstrate clinical benefit occurs rarely. For example, accelerated approval could be used for an acute condition where an effect on a surrogate endpoint could be shown in a small number of patients, but a much larger study would be needed to show the effect on a clinical outcome, such as survival.

FDA encourages sponsors to communicate with the Agency early in development concerning the potential eligibility of a drug for accelerated approval, proposed surrogate endpoints or intermediate clinical endpoints, clinical trial designs, and planning and conduct of confirmatory trials. A sponsor seeking accelerated approval may also need to prepare for a more rapid pace for other aspects of the drug development (e.g., manufacturing (see section IX.A.), development of a necessary companion diagnostic (see section IX.D.)).

A. Qualifying Criteria for Accelerated Approval

At the time a product is granted accelerated approval, FDA has determined that an effect on the endpoint used to support approval—a surrogate endpoint or an intermediate clinical endpoint—is reasonably likely to predict clinical benefit. The principal risk of this approach is the possibility that patients will be exposed to a drug that ultimately will not be shown to provide an actual clinical benefit. In addition, there generally will be fewer, smaller, or shorter clinical trials than is typical for a drug receiving traditional approval, which may generally mean there is less information about the occurrence of rare or delayed adverse events. Uncertainty about whether clinical benefit will be verified and the possibility of undiscovered risks are the primary reasons that accelerated approval is reserved for drugs intended to treat a serious condition and that appear to provide a meaningful advantage over available therapy.

1. Serious Condition

See section III.A.

2. Meaningful Advantage Over Available Therapy

The accelerated approval regulations state that accelerated approval is available only for drugs that provide a meaningful therapeutic benefit over existing treatments.[18] The accelerated approval provisions of section 901 of FDASIA (amending section 506 of the FD&C Act) require FDA to ". . .tak[e] into account . . . the availability or lack of alternative treatments."

Amended section 506(c) clarifies the Agency's flexibility in administering the accelerated approval program. For example, an alternative therapy with efficacy comparable to available therapy, but with a different mechanism of action, could be of added clinical value in a disease setting in which a significant number of patients may respond differently to the new therapy. The discussion of unmet medical need in section III.C.2. provides examples of situations in which a drug could be shown to provide a meaningful advantage over available therapy, including some in which there may not be a demonstrated direct efficacy or safety advantage.

Section III.B. describes what constitutes available therapy when determining whether a drug provides a meaningful advantage.

3. Demonstrates an Effect on an Endpoint That Is Reasonably Likely to Predict Clinical Benefit

These endpoints are discussed in section VII.B. The basis for determining whether an endpoint is reasonably likely to predict clinical benefit is discussed in section VII.C.

B. Accelerated Approval Endpoints

The two types of endpoints that can be used as a basis for accelerated approval are: (1) a surrogate endpoint that is considered reasonably likely to predict clinical benefit and (2) a clinical endpoint that can be measured earlier than IMM that is reasonably likely to predict an effect on IMM or other clinical benefit (also see section VII.D.2.). For purposes of this guidance, these categories of endpoints are referred to as surrogate endpoints and intermediate clinical endpoints, respectively.

A clinical endpoint is a characteristic or variable that directly measures a therapeutic effect of a drug—an effect on how a patient feels (e.g., symptom relief), functions (e.g., improved mobility), or survives.

A clinical benefit is a positive therapeutic effect that is clinically meaningful in the context of a given disease. The clinical benefit must be weighed against a treatment's risks to determine whether there is an overall benefit for patients (i.e., a positive benefit-risk profile).

1. Surrogate Endpoints

For purposes of accelerated approval, a surrogate endpoint is a marker, such as a laboratory measurement, radiographic image, physical sign, or other measure, that is thought to predict clinical benefit, but is not itself a measure of clinical benefit. Depending on the strength of the evidence supporting the ability of a marker to predict clinical benefit, the marker may be a surrogate endpoint that is known to predict clinical benefit (a validated surrogate endpoint that could be used for traditional approval), a surrogate endpoint that is reasonably likely to predict a drug's intended clinical benefit (and that could therefore be used as a basis for accelerated approval), or a marker for which there is insufficient evidence to support reliance on the marker as either kind of surrogate endpoint (and that therefore cannot be used to support traditional or accelerated approval of a marketing application).

Examples of surrogate endpoints that FDA has used to support accelerated approval include the following:

- Prolonged suppression of HIV viral load in plasma has been shown to reduce the morbidity and mortality associated with HIV disease and has been the basis for traditional approval. Shorter-term suppression of viral load has been used in the past as a surrogate to support accelerated approval because it was considered reasonably likely to predict an effect on morbidity or mortality. Data now demonstrate that short-term suppression of viral load may support full approval, in some circumstances.[19]

- Clearance of bacteria from the blood stream as evidenced by a laboratory measurement of bacteria in the blood has been considered reasonably likely to predict the clinical resolution of infection.
- Outcomes of 6-month follow-up treatment (i.e., sputum culture status and infection relapse rate) have been considered reasonably likely to predict the resolution of pulmonary tuberculosis.
- Decrease in iron stores for patients with iron overload caused by thalassemia has been considered reasonably likely to predict a decrease in transfusion-related adverse events caused by iron overload in the body.
- Radiographic evidence of tumor shrinkage (response rate) in certain cancer types has been considered reasonably likely to predict an improvement in overall survival.

2. Intermediate Clinical Endpoints

For purposes of accelerated approval, an intermediate clinical endpoint is a measurement of a therapeutic effect that can be measured earlier than an effect on IMM and is considered reasonably likely to predict the drug's effect on IMM or other clinical benefit. An important question is whether the demonstrated therapeutic effect alone would be a basis for traditional approval. Approvals for products for serious conditions based on clinical endpoints other than IMM will usually be considered under traditional approval procedures. Approvals based on such clinical endpoints will be considered under the accelerated approval pathway only when it is essential to determine effects on IMM or other clinical benefit in order to confirm the predicted clinical benefit that led to approval. Although FDA has limited experience with accelerated approvals based on intermediate clinical endpoints, FDA believes intermediate clinical endpoints generally could be used to support accelerated approval in situations such as:

- A study demonstrates a relatively short-term clinical benefit in a chronic disease setting in which assessing durability of the clinical benefit is essential for traditional approval, but the short-term benefit is considered reasonably likely to predict long-term benefit.
- A clinical endpoint demonstrates a clinical benefit that is reasonably likely to predict an effect on IMM in a disease setting in which it is

essential to confirm the effect on IMM (e.g., because available therapy has established effects on IMM).

Examples of cases in which FDA has used an intermediate clinical endpoint to support accelerated approval include the following:

- A treatment for multiple sclerosis was approved based on a large therapeutic effect on relapse rate through approximately 13 months of treatment, but where there was uncertainty about the durability of the observed effect. Under accelerated approval, the sponsor was required to continue the existing trials into the postmarketing period to confirm durability of the observed effect at 2 years.
- A treatment for preterm labor was approved based on a demonstration of delay in delivery. Under accelerated approval, the sponsor was required to conduct postmarketing studies to demonstrate improved long-term postnatal outcomes.

FDA will not grant accelerated approval to products that meet standards for traditional approval. Sponsors considering a development program for accelerated approval based on an intermediate clinical endpoint should discuss their development program with the appropriate review division early in drug development.

C. Evidentiary Criteria for Accelerated Approval

Drugs granted accelerated approval must meet the same statutory standards for safety and effectiveness as those granted traditional approval.[20] For effectiveness, the standard is substantial evidence based on adequate and well-controlled clinical investigations.[21] For safety, the standard is having sufficient information to determine whether the drug is safe for use under conditions prescribed, recommended, or suggested in the proposed labeling.[22] Under accelerated approval, FDA can rely on a particular kind of evidence, such as a drug's effect on a surrogate endpoint, as a basis for approval. FDA carefully evaluates such evidence to ensure that any remaining doubts about the relationship of the effect on the surrogate to clinical benefit are resolved by additional postapproval studies or trials.[23] An application for accelerated approval should also include evidence that a proposed surrogate endpoint or an intermediate clinical endpoint is reasonably likely to predict the intended clinical benefit of a drug.

Determining whether an endpoint is reasonably likely to predict clinical benefit is a matter of judgment that will depend on the biological plausibility of the relationship between the disease, the endpoint, and the desired effect and the empirical evidence to support that relationship. The empirical evidence may include ". . . epidemiological, pathophysiological, therapeutic, pharmacologic, or other evidence developed using biomarkers, for example, or other scientific methods or tools."[24] Evidence of pharmacologic activity alone is not sufficient, however.[25] Clinical data should be provided to support a conclusion that a relationship of an effect on the surrogate endpoint or intermediate clinical endpoint to an effect on the clinical outcome is reasonably likely.

In making the judgment as to whether a drug's effect on a given endpoint is reasonably likely to predict clinical benefit, FDA considers all relevant evidence and may consult external experts, as needed. This guidance provides an overview of some of the important factors to consider in identifying and assessing the predictive potential of surrogate endpoints or intermediate clinical endpoints. This guidance does not, however, address the specific clinical evidence needed to support a conclusion that a particular surrogate endpoint or intermediate clinical endpoint is reasonably likely to predict clinical benefit or IMM because such evidence is case-specific and is not readily generalizable.

1. Understanding of the Disease Process

Surrogate endpoints are often thought to be a measure of the following, for example:

- The underlying cause of the disease (e.g., elevated uric acid and gout, elevated blood pressure and hypertensive cardiovascular disease, low thyroxine levels and hypothyroidism, high ammonia levels and urea cycle disorders)
- An effect that predicts the ultimate outcome (e.g., tumor shrinkage could be expected to delay symptomatic progression and improve survival, diuresis could be expected to improve symptoms of heart failure, effects on serum creatinine or glomerular filtration rate (if not transient or reversible) are accepted surrogates for predicting effects on chronic renal disease and delaying the occurrence of end-stage renal disease)

- The state of the pathophysiologic pathway leading to the clinical outcome (e.g., low levels of the biomarker that increase with replacement of a missing enzyme or clotting factor)

In such cases, the extent to which the pathophysiology of a disease is understood is an important factor in determining whether an endpoint is reasonably likely to predict clinical benefit. If the disease process is complex, has multiple pathophysiologic or causal pathways, and is poorly understood, it may be difficult to determine whether an effect on a surrogate endpoint represents a meaningful effect on the causal pathway. For example, for some reasonably well-understood enzyme deficiencies, replacement of the deficient enzyme reliably predicts clinical benefit. In contrast, other enzyme deficiencies may involve a defect for which the pathophysiologic or causal pathways are not well understood and where enzyme replacement as measured by blood levels, but not tissue levels, will not reasonably predict the disease course or treatment results.

Some effects on well-established, disease-related biomarkers[26] may have little or no ability to predict clinical benefit or their ability to predict benefit may vary depending on the disease or the intervention. For example, in a patient with a fever caused by an infectious disease, a fall in a patient's body temperature in response to a non-steroidal anti-inflammatory drug does not predict the drug's effect on the disease. However, a fall in a patient's body temperature in response to an antibiotic may be an indication of an effect on the disease. Similarly, in prostate cancer, increased levels of prostate-specific antigen (PSA) may be the result of advancing tumor burden. Therefore, PSA may be correlated with the progression of prostate cancer and the risks of mortality. However, the relationship between increasing PSA and disease progression and morbidity is not uniform. Thus the ability of a drug to lower PSA levels cannot necessarily be relied upon to predict the drug's clinical benefit.

2. Understanding of the Relationship between the Drug's Effect and the Disease Process

The extent to which a drug's effect on the surrogate endpoint is known to predict an effect on the disease either because the effect is on the causal pathway or correlates with clinical outcomes is critical. Sometimes this relationship can be assessed epidemiologically but it is most persuasively established by knowing that a drug that affects the surrogate endpoint also affects a clinical outcome. Thus, lowering blood pressure has been shown repeatedly, with a wide variety of drugs, to reduce the incidence of stroke and cardiovascular disease in people with hypertension. Similarly, killing infecting bacteria or viruses leads to curing infectious disease and shrinking a tumor for a sustained period can lead to improved survival in patients with some cancers. These surrogate endpoint responses are thus understood to have positive effects on the disease process.

Examples of factors to consider in identifying and assessing a surrogate endpoint thus include the following:

- Whether there is reliable and consistent epidemiologic evidence supporting the relationship between the endpoint and the intended clinical benefit.[27]
- How precisely the epidemiologic relationship between the endpoint and clinical outcome is defined. For example, the extent to which an abnormal endpoint corresponds to a worse clinical outcome, as is the case for blood pressure and low-density lipoprotein (LDL) cholesterol. (The stronger the correlation between the abnormality and clinical outcome, the stronger the basis for concluding that an effect on the endpoint would have a reasonably well-defined effect on the clinical outcome.)
- Whether the effect on the surrogate endpoint has been shown to predict a clinical benefit with another drug or drugs. This factor would generally be more persuasive if the drug is in the same or a closely related pharmacological class.

Particularly in rare diseases, there may be limited information in the literature, lack of in-depth epidemiological or historical data, and little or no experience with other drugs to inform the interpretation of surrogate endpoints or intermediate clinical endpoints. FDA may consult with external experts on surrogate endpoints and intermediate clinical endpoints where there is a lack of historical data for a given disease.[28]

D. Conditions of Accelerated Approval

1. Promotional Materials

Unless otherwise informed by the Agency, an applicant must submit to the Agency for consideration during the preapproval review period copies of all promotional materials, including promotional labeling as well as advertisements, intended for dissemination or publication within 120 days following marketing approval.[29] After 120 days following marketing approval, unless otherwise informed by the Agency, the applicant must submit promotional materials at least 30 days prior to the intended time of initial dissemination of the labeling or initial publication of the advertisement.[30]

2. Confirmatory Trials

For drugs granted accelerated approval, postmarketing confirmatory trials have been required to verify and describe the anticipated effect on IMM or other clinical benefit. These trials must be completed with due diligence.[31]

FDA has interpreted the due diligence requirement to mean that the postmarketing trial(s) intended to verify the clinical benefit must be conducted promptly to facilitate determination, as soon as possible, of whether clinical benefit has been verified. The protocol for a postmarketing trial should be developed as early as possible, and timelines for the trial should be specified; for example, timelines for enrollment and trial completion should be stipulated. There should be agreement between FDA and the sponsor on the design and conduct of the confirmatory trial(s).

If it is clear during development that a product is intended to be approved under accelerated approval on the basis of a surrogate endpoint or an intermediate clinical endpoint, confirmatory trial(s) should be underway at the time the marketing application is submitted. If it is not clear until shortly before or after submission of a marketing application that a surrogate endpoint or an intermediate clinical endpoint will be the proposed basis for accelerated approval, there should be agreement on the design and conduct of such trial(s) before approval.

Generally, the confirmatory trial would evaluate a clinical endpoint that directly measures clinical benefit. For example, the confirmatory trial population would ordinarily be the same disease population that was studied to support accelerated approval. In some cases, however, the commercial availability of a drug following accelerated approval may make it difficult to enroll patients in the same disease population. In these cases, a confirmatory trial may be conducted in a different but related population that is capable of verifying the predicted clinical benefit. This is often the case in oncology, where after accelerated approval of a drug for late-stage disease is granted, the confirmatory trial is conducted in an earlier stage of the same cancer.

There are also cases in which additional evaluation (longer duration) of the same surrogate endpoint that was used to support accelerated approval (rather than a clinical endpoint) in the same population could be persuasive evidence of clinical benefit. For example, in the case of HIV treatment, an effect on viral load of relatively short duration (24 weeks) was considered reasonably likely to predict clinical benefit supporting accelerated approval. An effect of longer (1 year) viral load suppression was more convincingly related to durable clinical benefit in the setting of lifelong therapy and thus was used to verify clinical benefit for traditional approval.[32]

When it is possible to use a later effect in a trial to verify the effect seen earlier in the same trial that supported accelerated approval, the same clinical trial(s) can be used to support accelerated approval and verify and describe the clinical benefit. In this case, the protocol and the statistical analysis plan should clearly account for an analysis of the surrogate endpoint data to provide support for accelerated approval, with continuation of the randomized trial(s) to obtain data on the clinical endpoint that will be the basis for verifying the clinical benefit. When the same trial is used to support accelerated approval and verify clinical benefit, the data to verify the clinical benefit may be, in some cases, nearly complete by the time of accelerated approval.

3. Withdrawal of Accelerated Approval

FDA may withdraw approval of a drug or indication approved under the accelerated approval pathway if,[33] for example:

- A trial required to verify the predicted clinical benefit of the product fails to verify such benefit.
- Other evidence demonstrates that the product is not shown to be safe or effective under the conditions of use.
- The applicant fails to conduct any required postapproval trial of the drug with due diligence.
- The applicant disseminates false or misleading promotional materials relating to the product.

Approval of a drug may be withdrawn if trials fail to verify clinical benefit or do not demonstrate sufficient clinical benefit to justify the risks associated with the drug (e.g., show a significantly smaller magnitude or duration of benefit than was anticipated based on the observed effect on the surrogate).

If FDA determines there are grounds for withdrawal, the Agency may ask the applicant to request withdrawal of approval under § 314.150(d) or notify the applicant of FDA's proposal to withdraw approval in a notice of opportunity for hearing (NOOH). The NOOH generally will state the proposed grounds for withdrawal of approval.[34] Upon receipt of an NOOH, an applicant has 15 days to file a written request for a hearing. If an applicant does not request a hearing within 15 days, the applicant waives its opportunity for hearing.[35] An applicant may also request the Agency to withdraw approval of an application approved under accelerated approval.[36]

VIII. Priority Review Designation

An application for a drug will receive priority review designation if it is for a drug that treats a serious condition and, if approved, would provide a significant improvement in safety or effectiveness. In addition, specific statutory provisions provide for priority review for various types of applications, described in section IV. A priority designation is intended to direct overall attention and resources to the evaluation of such applications. This section describes the qualifying criteria and the features of priority review designation. Appendix 1 describes the process for priority review designation.

A. Qualifying Criteria for Priority Review Designation

1. Serious Condition

See section III.A.

2. Demonstrating the Potential to Be a Significant Improvement in Safety or Effectiveness

On a case-by-case basis, FDA determines at the time of NDA, BLA, or efficacy supplement filing whether the proposed drug would be a *significant improvement* in the safety or effectiveness of the treatment, prevention, or diagnosis of a serious condition. Significant improvement may be illustrated by the following examples:

- Evidence of increased effectiveness in treatment, prevention, or diagnosis of a condition
- Elimination or substantial reduction of a treatment-limiting adverse reaction
- Documented enhancement of patient compliance that is expected to lead to an improvement in serious outcomes
- Evidence of safety and effectiveness in a new subpopulation

Although such evidence can come from clinical trials comparing a marketed product with the investigational drug, a priority review designation can be based on other scientifically valid information. Generally, if there is an available therapy (see section III.B.), sponsors should compare their investigational drug to the available therapy in clinical testing with an attempt to show superiority relating to either safety or effectiveness. Alternatively, sponsors could show the drug's ability to effectively treat patients who are unable to tolerate, or whose disease failed to respond to, available therapy or show that the drug can be used effectively with other critical agents that cannot be combined with available therapy. Although such showings would usually be based on randomized trials, other types of controls could also be persuasive, for example, historical controls.[37]

B. Features of Priority Review Designation

A priority review designation means FDA's goal is to take action on the marketing application within 6 months of receipt (compared with 10 months under standard review). The PDUFA review clock for applications filed by FDA under the Program is described in section IV.

IX. General Considerations

Communication with the Agency is a critical aspect of expedited programs. FDA will strive to provide a timely response to a sponsor's inquiry regarding an expedited development program. It is equally critical that a sponsor respond promptly to FDA's inquiries.[38] This applies to formal meetings and related inquiries, written correspondence, and other interactions. In addition to the many types of formal meetings[39] and correspondence the Agency offers to sponsors, additional considerations for sponsors of expedited programs are highlighted in this section.

A. Manufacturing and Product Quality Considerations

The sponsor of a product that receives an expedited drug development designation may need to pursue a more rapid manufacturing development program to accommodate the accelerated pace of the clinical program. The sponsor's product quality and CMC teams should initiate early communication with FDA to ensure that the manufacturing development programs and timing of submissions meet the Agency's expectations for licensure or marketing approval.[40]

When sponsors receive an expedited drug development designation, they should be prepared to propose a commercial manufacturing program that will ensure availability of quality product at the time of approval. The proposal should consider estimated market demand and the commercial manufacturing development plan. The proposal should also consider manufacturing facilities and a lifecycle approach to process validation. Additionally, the proposal should include a timeline for development of the manufacturing capabilities with goals aligned with the clinical development program. After the initial discussion following designation, frequent communication during development will generally facilitate meeting manufacturing development goals and product quality goals.

Sponsors of such products should allow for an earlier submission of the CMC section (including product quality information) for timely review, and, critically, for inspection activities.[41] Coordination with the sponsor and contract manufacturers may be necessary to ensure that manufacturing facilities and equipment are ready for inspection during review of the clinical section of the application. A comprehensive meeting with FDA's product quality review groups in advance of submission may facilitate the quality assessment of products designated for expedited programs.

Although sponsors must ensure the availability of quality product at the time of approval, FDA may exercise some flexibility on the type and extent of manufacturing information that is expected at the time of submission and approval for certain components (e.g., stability updates, validation strategies, inspection planning, manufacturing scale-up). The level of flexibility will be determined on a case-by-case basis after consideration of factors such as the following: (1) product characteristics, (2) seriousness of the condition and medical need, (3) manufacturing processes, (4) the robustness of the sponsor's quality system, and (5) the strength of the sponsor's risk-based quality assessment. FDA's consideration of the sponsor's proposal for an integrated postmarketing plan will also take into account whether elements of the plan may be appropriately executed as a postmarketing commitment or requirement. For example, FDA will consider impacts on clinical performance, such as safety and immunogenicity. Sponsors should meet with the Agency to discuss their proposed plan as soon as possible and no later than the pre-NDA or pre-BLA meeting.

B. Nonclinical Considerations

To ensure timely submission and review of nonclinical data, sponsors should initiate early communication with FDA for their nonclinical study programs. Considerations such as study protocol modifications, sequence and scheduling of studies, and the need for specific studies (e.g., long-term toxicity) may be important in the context of expedited drug development. FDA will provide guidance to sponsors on the development of appropriate and timely nonclinical data needed to support an application for marketing approval or licensure.

C. Clinical Inspection Considerations

Sponsors should anticipate the Agency's need to inspect clinical trials, including, if applicable, the analytical component of bioavailability or bioequivalence studies. Sponsors should be prepared for inspections to be scheduled by the Agency early in the application review process so inspection results are available to inform the review division and to allow time for the sponsor to address significant inspection findings. To select sites for clinical inspections, it is important for reviewers to have timely access to adequate and accurate data in BLA, NDA, or supplement submissions. Sponsors should initiate early communication with FDA about information required for inspection planning and conduct.

D. Companion Diagnostics

Development programs utilizing one or more of the expedited programs described in this guidance may involve an in vitro companion diagnostic device. Sponsors using one of the expedited programs for a product that involves an in vitro companion diagnostic device should consult FDA's guidance on the topic.[42]

X. Paperwork Reduction Act of 1995

This guidance contains information collection provisions that are subject to review by the Office of Management and Budget (OMB) under the

Paperwork Reduction Act of 1995 (44 U.S.C. 3501-3520). The time required to complete this information collection is estimated to average 30 hours per response to prepare a priority review designation request, 70 hours per response to prepare a breakthrough therapy designation request, and 120 hours per request to prepare promotional materials for accelerated approval under § 314.550, including the time to review instructions, search existing data sources, gather the data needed, and complete and review the information collection. Send comments regarding this burden estimate or suggestions for reducing this burden to:

Food and Drug Administration
Center for Drug Evaluation and Research
Office of Medical Policy
10903 New Hampshire Avenue, Bldg. 51, rm. 6360
Silver Spring, MD 20993-0002

This guidance also refers to previously approved collections of information found in FDA regulations. The collections of information in 21 CFR 202.1, certain parts of part 314, part 601, and sections 506(b)(1), 735, and 736 of the FD&C Act have been approved under OMB control numbers 0910-0686, 0910-0001, 0910-0338, 0910-0389, and 0910-0297. An agency may not conduct or sponsor, and a person is not required to respond to, a collection of information unless it displays a currently valid OMB control number. The OMB control number for this information collection is 0910-0765 (expires 03/31/2017).

Appendix 1: Processes for Fast Track, Breakthrough Therapy, and Priority Review Designations

This appendix describes general processes applicable to the submission and review of fast track, breakthrough therapy, and priority review designations.

A. Process for Fast Track Designation

1. When to Send a Designation Submission

Sponsors may request fast track designation when the IND is first submitted or at any time thereafter before receiving marketing approval of their BLA or NDA. The IND and potential fast track designation may be discussed before an IND submission in a pre-IND meeting, but a decision on designation would await submission of the IND. As a practical matter, FDA should ordinarily receive a fast track designation request no later than the sponsor's pre-BLA or preNDA meeting with the Agency because many of the features of fast track designation will not apply after that time. If a sponsor's drug development program is granted fast track designation for one indication and has subsequently obtained data to support fast track designation for another indication, the sponsor should submit a separate request.

2. Where to Send a Designation Submission

The IND or amendment should be sent to the IND administrative file to the attention of the appropriate review division or office in CDER or CBER.

3. Content of a Designation Submission

Fast track designation requests should contain the following information (in most cases, this information could be captured in approximately 10 to 20 pages):

- If the fast track designation request is submitted to the sponsor's IND as an amendment, identification of the submission in the cover letter as a **REQUEST FOR FAST TRACK DESIGNATION** in bold, uppercase letters. If the request is submitted with an initial IND, identification of the submission in the cover letter as both an **INITIAL INVESTIGATIONAL NEW DRUG SUBMISSION** and **REQUEST FOR FAST TRACK DESIGNATION** in bold, uppercase letters.
- In the cover letter of the submission, the name of the sponsor's contact person and the contact person's address, email address, telephone number, and fax number.
- If applicable, the IND application number.

- If available, for drug products, the proprietary name and active ingredient and for biological products, the proper name and proprietary name.
- The division or office to which the IND is being submitted or in which it is active.
- The proposed indication(s).
- A concise summary of information that supports the fast track designation request for the indication being studied, including the following:
    - The basis for considering the drug to be one intended to treat a serious condition
    - The basis for considering the drug to have the potential to address an unmet medical need and an explanation of how this potential is being evaluated in the planned drug development program (e.g., a description of the trials intended to evaluate this potential)
- If applicable, a list of documents previously submitted to the IND that is considered relevant to the designation request, with reference to submission dates. Paper submissions can be resubmitted to FDA as appendices to the designation request.

4. FDA Response

FDA will respond to fast track designation requests within 60 calendar days of receipt of the request.

a. Designation Letter

If the Agency determines that the criteria for designation as a fast track drug development program have been met, the designation letter will:

- State that fast track designation is granted for development of the product for use in treating the specific serious condition
- Point out that the sponsor should design and perform studies that can show whether the product meets an unmet medical need
- Alert the sponsor to the need for the drug development program to continue to meet the criteria for fast track designation.

b. Nondesignation Letter

If the Agency determines that a fast track designation request was incomplete or that the drug development program failed to meet the criteria for fast track designation, the Agency will send a nondesignation letter to the sponsor. The nondesignation letter will state that fast track designation is not granted and explain the reasons for the Agency's decision.

5. Continued Designation as a Fast Track Development Program

Over the course of drug development, it can be expected that some products granted fast track designation will not continue to meet the criteria for fast track designation. A drug product in a fast track development program may not continue to meet the criteria if the drug: (1) no longer demonstrates a potential to address unmet medical need or (2) is not being studied in a manner that shows the drug product can treat a serious condition and meets an unmet medical need. The drug product may no longer demonstrate a potential to address unmet medical need, for example, if a new product was approved under a traditional approval that addressed the same need or if emerging clinical data failed to show that the product in a fast track development program had the anticipated advantage over available therapy. For products in fast track drug development programs, the Agency expects that the appropriateness of considering particular drug development plans as part of the fast track program will be discussed and evaluated during the drug development process, including at the end-of-phase 2 meeting and the pre-BLA or preNDA meeting. If the sponsor recognizes that the fast track drug development program will no longer be pursued, the sponsor should inform the Agency of this change.

When fast track designation is no longer supported by emerging data or the designated drug development program is no longer being pursued, the Agency may choose to send a letter notifying the sponsor that the program is no longer designated as a fast track drug development program.

B. Process for Breakthrough Therapy Designation

1. When to Send a Designation Submission

Although sponsors may request breakthrough therapy designation when the IND is first submitted or at any time thereafter, they should not send breakthrough therapy designation requests until they have preliminary clinical evidence indicating that ". . . the drug may demonstrate substantial improvement over existing therapies on 1 or more clinically significant endpoints."[43] FDA therefore expects that in most cases breakthrough therapy designation requests would be submitted as an amendment to the IND. Ideally,

FDA should receive a breakthrough therapy designation request before initiation of the clinical trial(s) intended to serve as the primary basis for demonstration of efficacy if most of the benefits of designation are to be obtained. Because the primary intent of breakthrough therapy designation is to develop evidence needed to support approval as efficiently as possible, FDA anticipates that breakthrough therapy designation requests will rarely be made after the submission of an original BLA or NDA or a supplement. If a sponsor's drug development program is granted breakthrough therapy designation for one indication and has subsequently obtained preliminary clinical evidence to support breakthrough therapy designation for another indication, the sponsor should submit a separate request.

If a sponsor has not requested breakthrough therapy designation, FDA may suggest that the sponsor consider submitting a request if: (1) after reviewing available data and information, the Agency thinks the drug development program may meet the criteria for breakthrough therapy designation and (2) the remaining drug development program and review can benefit from the designation. However, the Agency still needs to review the submitted request (including preliminary clinical evidence) to determine if it meets the criteria for breakthrough therapy designation. A suggestion by the Agency that a sponsor consider submitting a request for breakthrough therapy designation is advisory and should not be interpreted as guaranteeing breakthrough therapy designation once a request is submitted and reviewed.

2. Where to Send a Designation Submission

The IND or amendment should be submitted to the IND administrative file to the attention of the appropriate review division or office in CDER or CBER.

3. Content of a Designation Submission

Breakthrough therapy designation requests should contain the following information (in most cases, this information could be captured in approximately 10 to 20 pages):

- If the breakthrough therapy designation request is submitted to the sponsor's IND as an amendment, identification of the submission in the cover letter as a **REQUEST FOR BREAKTHROUGH THERAPY DESIGNATION** in bold, uppercase letters. If the request is submitted with an initial IND, identification of the submission in the cover letter as both an **INITIAL**

INVESTIGATIONAL NEW DRUG SUBMISSION and **REQUEST FOR BREAKTHROUGH THERAPY DESIGNATION** in bold, uppercase letters.

- In the cover letter of the submission, the name of the sponsor's contact person and the contact person's address, email address, telephone number, and fax number.
- If applicable, the IND application number.
- If available, for drug products, the proprietary name and active ingredient and for biological products, the proper name and proprietary name.
- The division or office to which the IND is being submitted or in which it is active.
- The proposed indication(s).
- A concise summary of information that supports the breakthrough therapy designation request for the indication being studied, including the following:
    - The basis for considering the drug to be one intended to treat a serious condition
    - The preliminary clinical evidence that the drug may demonstrate substantial improvement over available therapies.[44] FDA does not expect the sponsor to submit primary data (data sets); but, the sponsor should describe the preliminary clinical evidence, including, for example, a brief description of available therapies (if there are any) and their effectiveness; justification for the comparator selected for the clinical studies, the study design, the population studied, and the endpoint used; and a brief description of the study results and statistical analyses (including, for example, subgroup analysis).
- If applicable, a list of documents previously submitted to the IND that is considered relevant to the designation request, with reference to submission dates. Paper submissions can be resubmitted to FDA as appendices to the designation request.

4. FDA Response

FDA will respond to breakthrough therapy designation requests within 60 calendar days of receipt of the request.

a. Designation Letter

If the Agency determines that the criteria for designation as a breakthrough therapy development program have been met, the designation letter will:

- State that breakthrough therapy designation is granted for development of the product for use in treating the specific serious condition
- Explain that FDA will work closely with the sponsor to provide guidance on subsequent development, including providing advice on generating evidence needed to support the drug approval in an efficient manner
- Alert the sponsor to the need for the drug development program to continue to meet the criteria for breakthrough therapy designation

b. Nondesignation Letter

If the Agency determines that a breakthrough therapy designation request was incomplete or that the drug development program failed to meet the criteria for breakthrough therapy designation, the Agency will send a nondesignation letter to the sponsor. The nondesignation letter will state that a breakthrough therapy designation is not granted and explain the reasons for the Agency's decision. Where appropriate, the letter may also include advice to the sponsor regarding subsequent development, including what would be needed in a new breakthrough therapy designation request.

5. Continued Designation as a Breakthrough Therapy Development Program

Over the course of drug development, it can be expected that some products granted breakthrough therapy designation will no longer be considered a breakthrough therapy. For example, a drug development program may be granted breakthrough therapy designation using early clinical testing that shows a much higher response rate than available therapies. However, subsequent interim data derived from a larger study may show a response that is substantially smaller than the response seen in early clinical testing. Another example is where breakthrough therapy designation is granted to two drugs that are being developed for the same use. If one of the two drugs gains traditional approval, the other would not retain its designation unless its sponsor provided evidence that the drug may demonstrate substantial improvement over the recently approved drug. Additionally, if the sponsor recognizes that the development program designated as breakthrough therapy will no longer be pursued, the sponsor should inform the Agency of this change.

When breakthrough therapy designation is no longer supported by emerging data or the designated drug development program is no longer being pursued, the Agency may choose to send a letter notifying the sponsor that the program is no longer designated as a breakthrough therapy development program. Consistent with FDA's commitment to communicate frequently, and in an interactive manner, with sponsors of drugs designated as breakthrough therapies, FDA will notify the sponsor of its intent to rescind and will offer the sponsor an opportunity to justify its product's continued designation. FDA recognizes that sponsors of products that have had their breakthrough therapy designation rescinded because available data no longer support the designation may still have sufficient evidence after completion of the drug development program to support marketing approval.

C. Process for Priority Review Designation

FDA determines whether an application qualifies for priority review (versus standard review) for every application, not just when priority review is requested by the applicant. However, an applicant may expressly request priority review as described in the following sections.

1. When to Send a Designation Submission

Sponsors may request priority review designation when they submit an original BLA, NDA, or efficacy supplement. The Agency does not anticipate that priority review designation requests will be made after the filing of a BLA, NDA, or efficacy supplement.

2. Where to Send a Designation Submission

Priority review designation requests may be submitted with the original BLA, NDA, or efficacy supplement to the attention of the appropriate review division or office in CDER or CBER.

3. Content of a Designation Submission

Priority review designation requests should contain the following information:

- Identification of the submission in the cover letter as a **REQUEST FOR PRIORITY REVIEW DESIGNATION** in bold, uppercase letters.
- In the cover letter of the submission, the name of the sponsor's contact person and the contact person's address, email address, telephone number, and fax number.
- If available, for drug products, the proprietary name and active ingredient and for biological products, the proper name and proprietary name.
- The proposed indication(s).
- A concise summary of information that supports the priority review designation request, including the following:
  - The basis for considering the drug to be intended to treat a serious condition
  - The basis for the assertion that the drug would be a significant improvement in the safety or effectiveness of the treatment, prevention, or diagnosis of a serious condition

4. FDA Response

FDA will inform the applicant in writing of a priority review designation by day 60 of the review. The division will inform the applicant in writing of a standard review designation by day 74 of the review. Applications that are not filed do not receive a review designation.

5. Continued Priority Review Designation

After priority review designation is assigned, the timeline will not change during the first review cycle, even if a redetermination of review status is made because of approval of other drugs, availability of new data, or submission of a request for formal dispute resolution by the applicant. In addition, applications filed over protest are assigned a standard review. If the application is resubmitted after FDA's refuse-to-file decision or if the application is withdrawn before FDA's action and resubmitted, FDA will make its determination of review designation based on the resubmitted application.

Appendix 2: Processes for Rolling Review

This appendix describes general processes applicable to the submission and review of portions of an application, a feature of fast track designation (see section V.B.2.) and breakthrough therapy designation (see section V1.B.3.).

A. Agreement on Proposal

Sponsors obtain preliminary Agency agreement on the proposal at the pre-BLA or pre-NDA meeting or earlier for products with breakthrough therapy designation (e.g., end-of-phase 2 meeting). At the meeting, the sponsor and the review division should discuss: (1) the data that will be used to support effectiveness, (2) the schedule for submission of each portion of the BLA or NDA, and (3) a description of portions of the application to be submitted separately.

A request to submit portions of an application ordinarily should be included in the information package for the pre-BLA or pre-NDA meeting. If a sponsor seeks to submit portions of an application to the IND after the pre-BLA or pre-NDA meeting, the sponsor should make such a request and provide a proposed schedule for submission of portions of an application to the IND as soon as possible.

A request for submission of portions of an application should be sent as an amendment to the IND; attach Form FDA 1571. The amendment should be clearly identified as a **REQUEST FOR SUBMISSION OF PORTIONS OF AN APPLICATION** in bold, uppercase letters. FDA responds to sponsors' requests for submission of portions of an application by letter. FDA also responds to changes to an agreement to accept portions of an application by letter.

B. Portions of an Application Eligible for Early Submission

Generally, the Agency accepts for submission a complete section of a BLA or NDA only, such as the entire CMC section, toxicology section, or clinical section.[45] A section of a BLA or NDA should be submitted for review in a form adequate to have been included in a complete BLA or NDA submission. Drafts should not be included in a submission; if final reports need to be updated, the applicant should submit a formal amendment to the BLA or NDA with the revised information. Occasionally, the Agency may, in its discretion, accept less than a complete section if the Agency determines that such a subsection would constitute a reviewable unit and be useful in making the review process more efficient (e.g., less than a complete section could be a CMC section lacking final consistency lot data and long-term stability data, a toxicology section lacking chronic toxicology data, final study reports for some or all of the principal controlled trials without integrated summaries). The sponsor should confirm these subsections are final reports.

At the pre-BLA or pre-NDA meeting, the Agency and the sponsor should work together to clearly define the parameters of accepting an incomplete section and to determine whether FDA could conduct a meaningful review of the submission before receiving the missing information.

C. Submission of User Fees

A sponsor is required to pay applicable fees as stated in section 736 of the FD&C Act before FDA may commence review of any portion of an application. The applicant should submit Form FDA 3397 with applicable user fees and follow the same procedures as those followed when a complete application is submitted.

D. Commencement of Review

If FDA accepts a portion of an application, this does not necessarily mean that review will commence or proceed before the complete application is submitted. Actual commencement and scheduling of review depends on many factors, including staffing, workload, competing priorities, timeline for completing the application, and the perceived efficiency of commencing review before receipt of the complete submission.

E. Calculation of Review Time

The review clock will not begin until the applicant informs the Agency that a complete BLA or NDA was submitted.[46] After the Agency is notified of the complete application, we will make a filing determination within the usual time.[47]

Office of Communications
Division of Drug Information, WO51, Room 2201
Center for Drug Evaluation and Research
Food and Drug Administration
10903 New Hampshire Ave., Silver Spring, MD 20993
Phone: 301-796-3400; Fax: 301-847-8714
druginfo@fda.hhs.gov
http://www.fda.gov/Drugs/GuidanceComplianceRegulatoryInformation/Guidances/default.htm
and/or
Office of Communication, Outreach and Development
Center for Biologics Evaluation and Research
Food and Drug Administration
10903 New Hampshire Ave., WO71, Room 3128
Silver Spring, MD 20993
Phone: 800-835-4709 or 240-402-7800
ocod@fda.hhs.gov
http://www.fda.gov/BiologicsBloodVaccines/GuidanceComplianceRegulatoryInformation/Guidances/default.htm

End Notes

[1] This guidance has been prepared by the Center for Drug Evaluation and Research (CDER) in cooperation with the Center for Biologics Evaluation and Research (CBER) at the Food and Drug Administration.

[2] For the purposes of this guidance, all references to *drugs* or *drug products* include both human drugs and biological drug products regulated by CDER and CBER unless otherwise specified.

[3] Section III.A.1. explains that all references to serious conditions include life-threatening conditions.

[4] Food and Drug Administration, Interim Rule, Investigational New Drug, Antibiotic, and Biological Drug Product Regulations; Procedures for Drugs Intended to Treat Life-Threatening and Severely Debilitating Illnesses (53 FR 41516, October 21, 1988).

[5] Food and Drug Administration, Final Rule, New Drug, Antibiotic, and Biological Drug Product Regulations; Accelerated Approval (57 FR 58942, December 11, 1992) and Food and Drug Administration, Proposed Rule, New Drug, Antibiotic, and Biological Drug Product Regulations; Accelerated Approval (57 FR 13234, April 15, 1992).

[6] Part 312, subpart I.

[7] 21 CFR 312.300(b)(1).

[8] Sponsors considering an expedited drug development designation or program for a drug intended to avoid a serious adverse event associated with available therapy or diminish its severity should be aware that they will need to provide data that directly support the effect corresponding to the level of evidence needed to meet the qualifying criteria for the relevant designation or program (e.g., phase 3 data demonstrating lower incidence or severity of the serious adverse reaction compared to available therapy for priority review). The requisite data may be very difficult to obtain in early development, particularly for purposes of breakthrough therapy designation.

[9] There may be a substantial number of approved therapies with varying relevance to how a serious disease is currently treated in the United States, including therapies that are no longer used or are used rarely. Only in exceptional cases will a treatment that is not approved for the indicated use or is not FDA-regulated (e.g., surgery) be considered available therapy. In those cases, FDA may consider an unapproved or unlicensed therapy to constitute available therapy if the safety and effectiveness of the use is supported by compelling evidence, including extensive evidence in the published literature (e.g., certain well-established oncologic treatments).

[10] Section 506(d)(1) of the FD&C Act.

[11] After the sponsor completes the development program, the product may still have sufficient evidence to support marketing approval.

[12] We update guidances periodically. To make sure you have the most recent version of a guidance, check the FDA Drugs guidance Web page at http://www.fda.gov/Drugs/GuidanceComplianceRegulatoryInformation/Guidances/default.htm and the Biologics guidance Web page at http://www.fda.gov/BiologicsBloodVaccines/GuidanceComplianceRegulatoryInformation/Guidances/default.htm.

[13] Section 505(d) of the FD&C Act and section 351(a) of the Public Health Service Act.

[14] As noted in section IX., it is important that sponsors respond promptly to FDA inquiries, which may include, for example, requests for information on various aspects of the drug development program.

[15] For more discussion of alternative clinical trial designs, see the draft guidance for industry *Adaptive Design Clinical Trials for Drugs and Biologics* and the draft guidance for industry *Enrichment Strategies for Clinical Trials to Support Approval of Human Drugs and Biological Products.* When final, these guidances will represent FDA's current thinking on these topics. See also the ICH E10 and the guidance for clinical trial sponsors *Establishment and Operation of Clinical Trial Data Monitoring Committees.*

[16] Section 506(c)(2)(A) of the FD&C Act.

[17] Section 506(c)(1)(B) of the FD&C Act. 21 CFR 314.510 and 601.41 provide that the Agency may consider ". . . epidemiologic, therapeutic, pathophysiologic, or other evidence . . ." in determining whether an endpoint is reasonably likely to predict clinical benefit. FDASIA provides that FDA may consider ". . . epidemiological, pathophysiological, therapeutic, pharmacologic, or other evidence developed using biomarkers, for example, or other scientific methods or tools."

[18] 21 CFR 314.500 and 601.40.

[19] See the draft guidance for industry *Human Immunodeficiency Virus-1 Infection: Developing Antiretroviral Drugs for Treatment.* When final, this guidance will represent FDA's current thinking on this topic.

[20] Section 505(d) of the FD&C Act.

[21] Section 505(d)(5) of the FD&C Act.

[22] Section 505(d)(1) of the FD&C Act.

[23] 57 FR 58942 at 58948.

[24] Section 506(c)(1)(B) of the FD&C Act.

[25] 57 FR 58942.

[26] FDA's CDER has established the Biomarker Qualification Program to support work with external scientists and clinicians in developing biomarkers. The Biomarker Qualification Program offers a formal process to guide submitters as they develop biomarkers and rigorously evaluate them for use in the regulatory process. Details on the program are available at http://www.fda.gov/drugs/developmentapprovalprocess/drugdevelopmenttools qualificationprogram/ ucm284076.htm.

[27] Note, however, that such a relationship does not always predict a favorable effect, as illustrated by failure of drugs that effectively lower premature ventricular beat rates or raise high-density lipoprotein (HDL) cholesterol to have the expected cardiovascular benefits.

[28] See, for example, section 569(a)(2), (b), and (c) of the FD&C Act, *Consultation With External Experts on Rare Diseases, Targeted Therapies and Genetic Targeting of Treatments*, which describes general consideration for consultation with external experts, topics for consultation, and classification as special Government employees.

[29] 21 CFR 314.550 and 601.45.

[30] 21 CFR 314.550 and 601.45.

[31] Section 506(c)(3)(A) of the FD&C Act and §§ 314.510 and 601.41. Where confirmatory trials verify clinical benefit, FDA generally will terminate the requirement (21 CFR 312.560 and 601.46).

[32] Although an effect on viral load changes of short duration had been used in the past as a surrogate endpoint to support accelerated approval, FDA now considers this endpoint acceptable, in some circumstances, to grant traditional approval based on years of experience with this endpoint.

[33] See section 506(c)(3) of the FD&C Act and §§ 314.530(a) and 601.43(a). Part 314, subpart E and part 601, subpart H describe additional grounds for withdrawal.

[34] 21 CFR 314.530(b) and 601.43(b).

[35] 21 CFR 314.530(c)(1) and 601.43(c)(1).

[36] 21 CFR 314.150(c) and 601.5(a).

[37] Sponsors contemplating the use of historical controls should consult ICH E10 for more-detailed discussions.

[38] For example, FDA may request updates on a breakthrough therapy designation program in order to provide the sponsor with guidance on drug development.

[39] See the guidance for industry *Formal Meetings Between the FDA and Sponsors or Applicants*. Also see the *CDER 21st Century Review Process Desk Reference Guide* accessible at http://www.fda.gov/downloads/AboutFDA/CentersOffices/CDER/ManualofPoliciesProced ures/UCM218757.htm.

[40] See the guidance for industry *IND Meetings for Human Drugs and Biologics Chemistry, Manufacturing, and Controls Information*.

[41] For products designated as fast track or breakthrough therapy, this can be accomplished through rolling review (see section V.B.2., section VI.B.3., and Appendix 2). For products submitted under an NDA without such a designation, flexibility is permitted in § 314.50(d)(1)(iv). For BLAs without such a designation, there is flexibility also to allow an early submission of the CMC section when resources permit.

[42] See the draft guidance for industry and Food and Drug Administration staff *In Vitro Companion Diagnostic Devices*. When final, this guidance will represent the FDA's current thinking on this topic.

[43] Section 506(a)(1) of the FD&C Act.

[44] If the designation is being submitted with the IND, examples of information that could be submitted to support a designation request include data from foreign clinical trials not conducted under IND, a different formulation or route of administration, a use in an unrelated indication, or the published literature.

[45] Form FDA 356h may be a useful guide to items in a BLA or NDA.

[46] Section 506(d)(2) of the FD&C Act provides that any time period for review of human drug applications shall not apply until the date on which the application is complete.

[47] See § 314.101, CDER MAPP 6025.4, *Good Review Practice: Refuse to File*, available on the Internet at http://www.fda.gov/downloads/aboutfda/centersoffices/officeofmedicalproducts andtobacco/cder/manualofpoliciespr ocedures/ucm370948.htm and CBER SOPP 8404, *Refusal to File Procedures for Biologic License Applications* (August 27, 2007), available on the Internet at http://www.fda.gov/BiologicsBloodVaccines/GuidanceCompliance RegulatoryInformation/ProceduresSOPPs/ucm07 3474.htm.

INDEX

D

E

F

G

H

I

L

M

N

O

P

R